*New Hope
for Problem
Pregnancies*

The purpose of this book is to make you aware of the normal progress of pregnancy and the possible ways in which it may go awry. The assessment of symptoms requires an expert. Proper diagnosis and therapy of all symptoms connected with pregnancy call for careful attention to your concerns by your doctor.

New Hope for Problem Pregnancies

Helping Babies BEFORE They're Born

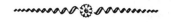

by Dianne Hales
& Robert K. Creasy, M.D.

Introduction by Arthur J. Salisbury, M.D.,
Vice-President for Medical Services,
March of Dimes Birth Defects Foundation

HARPER & ROW, PUBLISHERS, New York
Cambridge, Philadelphia, San Francisco, London
Mexico City, São Paulo, Sydney

1817

For my parents, with love

D.H.

FIRST EDITION

Designed by Ruth Bornschlegel

Library of Congress Cataloging in Publication Data

Hales, Dianne R., 1950–
  New hope for problem pregnancies.

  Bibliography: p.
  Includes index.
  1. Pregnancy, Complications of. 2. Prenatal diagnosis. 3. Prenatal care. I. Creasy, Robert K. II. Title.
RG571.H29 1982   618.3   81–47657
ISBN 0-06-014934-5   AACR2

---

82 83 84 85 86 10 9 8 7 6 5 4 3 2 1

Contents

v

APPENDIXES

Acknowledgments

The idea for this book grew out of several articles we worked together on about high-risk pregnancies. It could not have become a reality without the support and help of many people at the University of California, San Francisco (UCSF). We are grateful to Drs. Julian Parer, James Roberts, Russell Laros, and Barry Block of UCSF's Department of Reproductive Sciences; to Dr. Mitchell Golbus for his consultations on genetics and drug risks; to Dr. Michael Katz for his many contributions to the book's organization and contents; to Helen Rizzo, R.N., and Marie Herron, R.N., for their invaluable assistance and enthusiastic cooperation; to Barbara Abrams for her help in preparing the information on nutrition; to Bonnie Gradstein, Libby Colman, and the obstetrical social workers for their insights on the psychological aspects of problem pregnancies; and to Valerie Briscoe, R.N., and the nurses of the delivery room and intensive care nursery at UCSF. We owe a special debt to Michela Reichman of UCSF's News and Public Information Office; William Burgower of J. B. Lippincott; Dr. Richard Depp of Northwestern University School of Medicine, who provided a comprehensive and helpful critique of the manuscript; and to our editor, Ann Harris, who shaped and polished it. We would also like to thank the dozens of women who shared their experiences with us and talked freely and openly about their own pregnancies in the hope that they could help other women in similar situations.

The writing of this book took place over many months and many thousands of miles, from Carmel to Cornwall. Through it all, Dr. Robert Hales provided constant encouragement and loving support—invaluable contributions to the book's development and completion.

Preface

This is a book that at first glance might seem scary, since it is filled with things that can go wrong during pregnancy. It deals not with the ideal circumstances of every expectant mother's fantasy, but with her deepest fear: that something, somehow may jeopardize the well-being or survival of her unborn baby.

However, we have written this book to inform rather than alarm, to point out that the prospects for having a healthy baby are better today than ever before. Yes, there are risks and problems in pregnancy—as there always have been. But for too long there's been an uneasy silence about them. Some women, fearful of finding out too much, have lived with the dread that comes of knowing too little.

New Hope for Problem Pregnancies shatters the long silence about the most precarious times of a life—the months before and the moment of birth. It provides the data, descriptions, and understanding that you'll need in order to recognize and try to overcome risks to your unborn baby. It is, in part, a report from one of medicine's most exciting frontiers, one that can help you understand the advances that are helping to save babies before birth. Since the technology of modern obstetrics can be intimidating, it describes procedures in detail, along with the reasons each is performed, the risks involved, and what the mother will see and feel.

This book goes beyond discussing what doctors can do to save babies to explain what mothers can do to protect and help their unborn children. We've included information on nutrition, exercise, the risks and benefits of drugs, the reasons for the absolute necessity of regular prenatal care. We explain in detail the special precautions some high-risk mothers may have to take, but our focus is on helping mothers to feel and act like participants, rather than patients. And since pregnancy involves not just the womb but the entire woman, we've tried to provide a mother's-eye view of nine of the most challenging months of a lifetime. We present medical information in the personal context of what mothers-to-be experience on the way to delivery. And we deal with psychological as well as physiological experiences, such as the unique emotional demands of coping with a complicated pregnancy or of losing a baby before or shortly after delivery.

We believe that the more you know about what is happening to your body and about the way your baby is developing, the more you'll be able to do—for yourself and your baby. But no book can be a substitute for a close, trusting relationship with your obstetrician. Only your doctor can evaluate the specific circumstances of your pregnancy and take into account all the variables affecting you and your baby. It always is important to choose an obstetrician you trust; in a complicated pregnancy, such trust is critical. You, your doctor, and other specialists in perinatal medicine should work as a team toward the common goal of giving your baby a healthy start in life. This book may answer some of your questions. It also should motivate you to ask other questions of your own doctor, who may take a somewhat different approach to specific problems or choose alternatives more suited to you and your baby's unique needs.

There is indeed new hope for mothers and babies at risk—if they get the special care they need before birth. This book can be the first step in recognizing and overcoming the risks to your baby. We hope that, as part of a much larger nationwide effort to help babies before they're born, it helps you and all of today's mothers give tomorrow's children the best possible future.

Introduction

Most women who become pregnant can look forward to nine months of joyful expectation with only slight discomforts and changes in lifestyle. With prenatal care obtained early and regularly, this forecast for most women will prove correct.

In about 20 percent of pregnancies, however, the course is not perfectly smooth. It is often possible to determine that problems may arise because of the woman's previous medical or obstetrical history. These cases are usually classified as "high risk," but that term often exaggerates the gravity of the situation. Other women may begin a pregnancy with no indications that problems will arise, but warning signals appear later, usually in the middle or late months. These cases then move to the "high risk" classification. Unsatisfactory as this term is, it means that these women must have special attention if they and their babies are to continue safely through the pregnancy and the delivery.

This book deals with the subject of these problem pregnancies. It is a book of hope and encouragement. Most of it could not have been written ten years ago because the knowledge of cause, diagnosis, and treatment of many abnormalities of pregnancy has been developed in the past decade. With this knowledge, it is possible for physicians to determine the condition of both patients involved in a pregnancy, the mother and baby, and to undertake treatment to produce a healthy outcome for both.

Knowing that help is available should relieve the anxieties of women who must have special attention during pregnancy. The relief of apprehension is important in treating problem pregnancies, and that is what this book is intended to do. The information given in this book will also prepare women to join physicians and nurses as partners in their own care.

Arthur J. Salisbury, M.D.,
Vice-President for Medical Services,
March of Dimes Birth Defects Foundation

The history of the nine months preceding . . . birth would probably be far more interesting and contain events of greater moment than all the three score and ten years that follow it.

SAMUEL TAYLOR COLERIDGE

PART 1

A Healthy Beginning

1 . The Era of the Fetus

JULIA ANN HALL YAWNS mightily at the end of a most remarkable day—her very first. Her mother rubs a finger along her new daughter's cheek. Like a kitten, Julia lifts her chin, her mouth working silently, her breathing as even as a purr. While her parents watch in awed delight, she stretches and settles into sleep.

This might seem like the most ordinary of scenes, acted out by hundreds of new families every day. Yet this baby truly is extraordinary. To the Halls, Julia is the child they feared they never could have. And to the physicians who specialize in caring for mothers and babies in the perinatal period—the time before, during, and immediately after birth—Julia is a living symbol of the progress they've made in saving babies before they're born.

For a long time Julia's parents had felt that they shouldn't dare to attempt another pregnancy. They remembered their first child, born too soon, too small, and too sick to survive. The neonatologists—pediatricians who specialize in caring for sick babies in their first days of life—had done their very best for the little boy born more than three months before his expected arrival date. But it was not enough to save his life.

Yearning for a child, the Halls worried about another preterm birth and another wrenching loss. They decided to try again only when their obstetrician told them about new approaches to the problem of preterm labor. This time Julia's mother learned how to detect the subtle signs of too-early contractions. When she became suspicious, she sought immediate treatment. As a result, Julia was able to get all the time she needed to prepare for birth.

Stories like Julia's are unusual but not uncommon. Each year some 3,700,000 women in the United States give birth. Most of their pregnancies are uneventful, most of their deliveries uncomplicated, and

3

most of their newborns healthy. But the fantasy of *all* pregnancies and deliveries being safe and simple is exactly that—a wish, not a reality. Nature can, and all too often does, falter. In about 10 to 15 percent of pregnancies, there is a significantly increased risk of a problem; in as many as 30 to 40 percent, there is some exception to the usual course of development and delivery. Rarely is the mother herself endangered; the life at stake is usually that of the unborn baby.

The possible risks to a fetus include genetic disorders, exposure to harmful chemicals, poor nutrition, infection, maternal diseases, and complications during pregnancy and delivery. The toll these dangers take is high: some 500,000 potential lives lost in miscarriages and still-births each year; more than 250,000 babies born with defects that may affect all the days of their lives. The total number of deaths and injuries each year is greater than that for children *and* adults killed in accidents of every type. Yet many of these babies could be saved or spared lifelong impairment, if they were given special attention and care while still in their mother's wombs.

Until quite recently very little was known about life before birth or about what could go wrong in pregnancy and why, so very little could be done to prevent these problems. But in the past twenty years a new approach to problems in pregnancy, called maternal-fetal medicine or perinatology, has emerged. Today perinatologists, working with mothers at risk, are rewriting the life stories of thousands of babies, changing almost-certain tragedies into tales of hope and triumph. This book is about such stories, about babies like Julia whose lives are jeopardized before they begin, and about the continuing struggle to give all babies the best possible start in life.

The concept of caring for a baby before birth represents a major change in medical thinking. Previously, obstetricians concentrated on the patient they could see, touch, and treat: the mother-to-be. Their improved understanding of how pregnancy affects a woman's health helped reduce the maternal mortality rate to a fraction of what it had been in prior decades. But the fetus, viewed more as a passenger than a patient, long remained a biological mystery. How could physicians attempt to treat an unborn baby when they couldn't examine it? How could they meet the needs of both patients without creating risks for either the baby or the mother?

Less than a generation ago, medical scientists developed a tool that could provide some answers to such questions. That technique—the first prenatal diagnostic test—was amniocentesis, a method of sampling the amniotic fluid that surrounds a fetus in order to obtain clues about its well-being. Other pioneering diagnostic procedures for the unborn include innovations such as sound waves that produce images of the fetus, biochemical tests of key proteins in the mother's blood and urine, and a still-experimental method of peering directly into the womb. With these tools obstetricians today can find out more about an unborn baby than would have been thought possible thirty years ago.

As physicians have learned more about life before birth, the fetus has emerged as a patient in its own right. It has become clear that the nine months of pregnancy can determine whether a baby is healthy at birth, develops normally as a child, and reaches full potential as an adult. It also is clear that the time to save lives and prevent impairment is before, as well as after, a baby is born. And with new understanding, new skills, and new optimism, that is exactly what perinatologists have set out to do.

One of their most dramatic successes would be remarkable in any field of medicine: the conquest of a major health threat in the course of a single generation. The problem, which once annually claimed 10,000 lives before or after birth and caused mental retardation in 20,000 infants who survived, was Rh disease. In the 1940s, scientists identified a blood component, which they called the Rh factor, that could be found in most, but not all, Americans. They observed that if the blood of an Rh-negative woman (one who did not have this substance) mingled with the blood of an Rh-positive baby she had conceived, her body would produce protective antibodies. Though her first baby would be healthy, in a subsequent pregnancy these antibodies would attack the blood cells of the Rh-positive baby she was carrying, endangering its life.

With new insight into this problem, physicians devised an effective treatment: transfusions of red blood cells directly to the fetus. This delicate procedure helped save the lives of thousands of babies at risk. Then in the 1960s a better alternative was found, a means of preventing the very formation of these destructive antibodies. Today far fewer pregnancies are complicated by this danger, and perinatal deaths related to Rh problems are uncommon.

Striking progress also has been made against rubella (German measles), another killer and crippler of the unborn. The symptoms of this viral infection are so mild in adults that rubella wasn't considered dangerous in pregnancy until a few decades ago. In 1964–65, a rubella epidemic swept the United States, leaving more than 20,000 babies of mothers who had been exposed to the virus with vision problems, hearing loss, heart malformations, and mental retardation. This outbreak, a tragedy for the babies and their families, was an opportunity for medical research. In 1966 scientists developed a quick, easy test for determining whether a mother-to-be is immune to rubella. In 1969 they produced a vaccine that can protect a susceptible woman and any children she conceives. However, rubella remains a potential threat, for an estimated 10 to 15 percent of all women of child-bearing age have not yet been immunized against it.

At birth, the most vulnerable babies of all are the littlest, those who weigh less than 2,500 grams (5½ pounds). Only 15 to 20 percent of all infants have such low birth weights, but they account for more than half of perinatal deaths. Once all babies this small were thought to have been born too soon, but physicians have discovered that as many as 40 percent are mature but, because of growth problems in the womb, small for their gestational age (SGA). The distinction between premature and SGA babies has proved to be significant, for the two groups encounter different problems before, during, and after birth. Understanding these difficulties has helped perinatologists cope with the big problems facing many small babies.

The primary threat for those babies at risk of being born prematurely is arriving in the world before they are physiologically capable of surviving in it. Smaller and smaller and younger and younger babies have been saved in the past two decades, but prematurity still remains the greatest problem in modern obstetrics. While new drugs are available to help buy more time in the womb, they are effective only if used very early in labor. If delivery cannot be delayed for more than a few days, perinatologists now have another option: they can give the mother injections of steroids, powerful drugs that speed up her baby's lung development and reduce its risk of having breathing problems after birth.

SGA babies face a different threat at a different time. Unable to get the nutrients and oxygen they need, they are at considerably greater risk of dying *before* birth. Obstetricians have to balance the dangers to the baby within the womb with the possible risks of a too-early delivery. Using new testing methods, they can monitor a baby's condition and schedule delivery for a time that will give the too-small infant the best possible chance of survival.

There also has been progress in assuring more women with chronic medical problems, such as diabetes, of successful pregnancies. For a long time the incidence of perinatal deaths for diabetic mothers was much higher than usual. More babies' lives have been saved in recent decades, but the incidence of birth defects in the babies of diabetics has remained disturbingly high. Nonetheless, years of research into the ways in which pregnancy affects metabolism and in which metabolic disorders like diabetes affect pregnancy are beginning to pay off. Diabetic women who plan their pregnancies carefully and maintain good metabolic control from the start now have an excellent chance of having healthy, normal babies.

In problems like diabetes, proper treatment for the mother is essential in assuring the well-being of her unborn baby. But when the fetus is the one with the disorder, perinatologists have to take another approach. Often they treat the mother as a way of indirectly caring for her baby. In California, for example, an unborn baby was diagnosed as suffering from a potentially lethal lack of biotin, a key vitamin. Each day throughout her pregnancy, the mother was given a supplement of biotin; at birth her baby was healthy and strong. In other circumstances, surgeons have performed delicate operations directly on the unborn to correct defects such as hydrocephalus (excessive fluid within the skull) and obstruction of the fetal bladder. Such still-experimental surgery before birth—which would have boggled the imagination a few years ago—may improve a baby's chance of survival and prevent permanent damage.

Other methods of protecting the unborn are less dramatic but equally significant. Ever since the 1960s, when the birth of thousands of babies with limb deformities alerted the world to the dangers of the sedative thalidomide, there has been greater restraint in the use of drugs in pregnancy. More prescription and nonprescription medications, as well as such commonly used—and abused—substances as alcohol and cigarettes, have been added to the list of suspected threats to a baby's health. Now physicians weigh the potential benefits of any drug given to the mother against its possible risk to the developing fetus.

One continuing challenge for everyone concerned with saving babies is making perinatal care available to *all* pregnant women. Most of the experts in this relatively new field are at major medical centers, as is the complex and extremely expensive technology needed to diagnose and treat babies before birth. While a relatively high percentage of pregnant women around the country encounter some risks, the number of mothers-to-be requiring special care in any one geographical area is usually too small to justify the costs of a perinatal center. And so health-care providers have taken a different approach to guaranteeing access to perinatal services: regionalization.

In the mid-1970s the country was divided into geographic regions in order to improve health care and reduce costly duplication of services. Each region contains a major perinatal center that can provide all necessary services, as well as hospitals capable of handling some, but not all, pregnancy complications, and smaller rural hospitals. An outreach consultation and education program fosters close cooperation among the area's physicians and hospitals. To work together efficiently, hospitals and doctors use standard forms and records. If long distances separate patients from the specialists at perinatal centers, transportation systems—including ambulances, helicopters, and planes—become an integral part of the program. The initial evaluations of the first regional systems have shown declines of 30 to 42 percent in newborn mortality rates.

What all this means to you, if you encounter problems in your pregnancy, is the promise of the best possible care when you need it most, regardless of where you live. You may never have any direct contact with perinatologists several hundred miles away, but your obstetrician may consult with them every week or every month. If necessary, you may visit a specially equipped hospital periodically for various tests during your pregnancy. And if there is any possibility that you or your baby will need extra care during or after delivery, you may be transferred to a perinatal center before labor begins.

An excellent indicator of the impact of this commitment to the unborn and newborn is the improved survival rate for American infants. From World War II to the 1960s, the newborn mortality rate in the U.S. was quite high compared with that of other industrialized nations: 35 deaths for every 1,000 live births. In 1981 our national mortality rate for newborns was lower than ever before: approximately 12 deaths per 1,000 births. In some regions, primarily those in which pregnant women have ready access to prenatal care and perinatal services, only 6 or 7 of every 1,000 babies died in the first month of life. More than 98 percent of infants survived the first—and most precarious—year of their lives.

Perinatologists have been able to save more lives because they've crossed the frontier of birth to intervene before babies enter the world. This step, and their success, is indeed impressive, but the months of pregnancy still remain largely unexplored territory. Scientists may know more than ever before about life's earliest days, but questions still outnumber answers. Physicians may be able to do more to safeguard mothers and their babies, but they cannot anticipate or prevent every possible problem. The best solutions available for some problems are merely stopgap measures buying time until the development of a better therapy or a means of prevention.

But while a great deal of perinatology is new and pioneering, its fundamental goal is timeless, one shared by all expectant mothers of the past, present, and future: to do everything that can be done for a baby beginning its life. The right to be "well-born," to inherit a legacy of good health and the potential for a long, full life, is the most basic of birthrights—and the most difficult to guarantee.

In the coming years science will undoubtedly provide more insights into the unique needs of babies preparing for life. Meeting those needs will demand the best in medical research, technology, and practice. It also will demand a willingness on the part of future parents to take on the responsibilities of parenting even before they see their children and to forge working partnerships with perinatologists for the sake of preventing as well as correcting problems in and after pregnancy.

Perinatology may well be the ultimate form of preventive medicine. In no other medical specialty can early detection of risks and preventive measures have such a profound impact over such a prolonged period of time. It certainly isn't unusual for a life to hang in the balance in any medical endeavor. But in perinatology there is a critical difference: what is at stake is not simply a life, but a lifetime.

2 . Nine Months of Changes

MARYANN BRANLEY CLOSES her eyes and falls back on the pillow. It has happened again—a sudden queasiness as she rose from the bed. She lies still, waiting for the wave of nausea to subside. This is the fifth day that she's awakened with an odd sensation in her stomach. Her breasts are tender and sore; her menstrual period is almost ten days overdue.

Wondering if she might be pregnant, Maryann thinks back, counting days, remembering nights. "You should be able to know the moment it happens," she says to herself, "to realize right from the start that you're going to have a baby." But her mind stays in the past only briefly, as she begins to count forward to the time when her baby might be born. She fantasizes about the future, about a child a little like her and a little like Mark, about an infant to hold and love. She smiles, rubbing a hand over her flat stomach and speculating about what she might look like in a month, or two months, or six. "Well," she says out loud, "I guess I'll just have to wait and see."

For every mother-to-be, pregnancy involves nine months of waiting and seeing. It is an experience unlike any other, crowded with changes and surprises. Every part of it can be astonishing, even to the woman who has had several children. All pregnancies have common characteristics and predictable patterns, but none is exactly like any other.

In the course of building your baby, your body will change in many ways—some obvious, some subtle, some startling, some unsettling. After years of not growing very much in any direction, it may be alarming to see so many changes happening so fast. You may feel that you are both the main character in an ongoing drama and a member of the audience watching the plot unfold. After all, every pregnancy does involve two stories: the story of the woman who conceives and carries the baby and the story of the new life taking form within her.

In order to get a preview of how your body may change and how

10

your baby will grow, let's follow the course of Maryann's pregnancy. Her story and that of the person who someday would be known as Matthew Branley may help you anticipate the normal changes of pregnancy and understand why they occur.

· Becoming a Mother

Like many women, Maryann didn't have to be told she was pregnant; her body gave her the first clues. Even before she had missed a menstrual period, she had felt a fullness in her breasts, an uneasiness in her stomach, and overwhelming fatigue late in the day. The changes were similar to her feelings just before a period, but more intense and persistent.

In a typical menstrual cycle, one of Maryann's ovaries would release an ovum, or egg cell, about two weeks after the first day of her last period. Her ovaries would secrete the hormone progesterone to prepare the lining of her uterus for a possible pregnancy. If the egg was not fertilized, the manufacture of progresterone would stop, and the uterine lining would be shed as a menstrual period.

This month was different, however. At the midpoint of Maryann's menstrual cycle, her ovary released one of its stored eggs. During intercourse her husband, Mark, ejaculated several million sperm into her vagina. Millions were destroyed on the perilous route from her vagina through her cervix, up her uterus, and into the fallopian tubes. Millions swam up the wrong tube. But all that was necessary was that one sperm cell find the right way at the right time. When that one sperm penetrated the cell membrane of Maryann's ovum, the remarkable process of development that would culminate in Matthew Branley's birth began.

By the time Maryann began to suspect that she was pregnant, the fertilized egg had multiplied into a cluster of cells and had floated down her fallopian tube to imbed itself in the wall of her uterus. Little fingerlike projections called villi burrowed into her uterine blood supply. These villi produced a chemical messenger to signal her ovaries to continue their output of progesterone. This messenger substance, called human chorionic gonadotropin (HCG), appears in a woman's body only in pregnancy. The detection of HCG in Maryann's urine—first in a home test, then in a laboratory analysis—confirmed that she was indeed pregnant. And on examination her doctor noted certain significant internal changes: her uterus was slightly larger; and her cervix was softer and appeared blue because of the increased blood flow to it.

The high levels of HCG produced during the first three months (trimester) were responsible for some of Maryann's discomforts in early pregnancy. Progesterone and estrogen triggered changes in the milk glands and ducts in her breasts, so they increased in size and felt somewhat tender. The pressure of the growing uterus against the bladder caused a more frequent need to urinate. But for Maryann, as for many women, the changes of the first trimester were exactly that: slight variations in the way she normally felt and acted.

The midtrimester—the fourth through the sixth month—was a quiet time for Maryann. She felt more energetic and calmer than before, but the transformation of her body became much more noticeable. Her waistline disappeared; her breasts became fuller; her stomach was round and firm. The skin around her nipples, the areola, darkened. She also noticed a dark line, called the linea nigra, down the center of her abdomen and a masklike darkening of the pigment in her cheeks. Her vaginal secretions increased, and Maryann sensed that she was sweating and salivating more than usual. She developed yearnings for odd foods—not just the stereotyped pickles and ice cream, but exotic dishes she'd never liked before.

Some of the most dramatic changes weren't visible in Maryann's periodic self-inspections. By the end of the sixth month, her uterus had increased its weight by twenty times. The production of blood cells in her body had accelerated, and her total blood volume had increased by 30 to 50 percent. Her heart, working harder to pump the greater supply of blood, enlarged slightly and shifted its position. By midpregnancy her breasts, functionally ready for nursing, began to secrete a thin amber or yellow substance called colostrum.

The most exciting experience came in Maryann's fifth month, when she began to feel her baby moving within her. At first she couldn't be sure if the vague sensations in her stomach were kicks or cramps. But as the baby's movements increased, its activity became unmistakable. Maryann would lie in bed at night, holding Mark's hand over her stomach, waiting for the prods and pokes that made their baby seem real and added to their sense of anticipation.

By the final three months of her pregnancy, Maryann was feeling more uncomfortable. As her belly grew, Maryann joked about "the body she used to own." Her growing uterus pushed against her lungs, and she became breathless after even a short walk. Yet in actuality her chest cage had widened, and she was breathing in more oxygen than usual. The pressure of her uterus made it more difficult for the veins of her lower limbs to empty; her legs and ankles would become swollen if she spent too many hours on her feet, particularly in warm weather. As her uterus squeezed against her stomach, digestive acid was pushed into her esophagus, causing heartburn.

In her ninth month, Maryann would stand before her mirror and marvel at the changes pregnancy had brought. Once her baby "dropped," or settled low in her pelvis, she found breathing much easi-

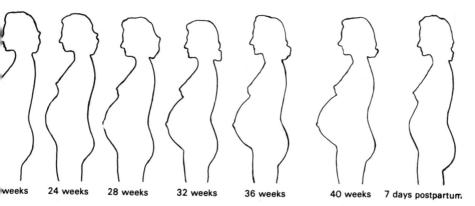

weeks   24 weeks   28 weeks   32 weeks   36 weeks   40 weeks   7 days postpartum.

Normal changes in abdominal contour in pregnancy *(from Reeder, Mastroianni, and Martin,* Maternity Nursing, *14th ed. J. B. Lippincott, 1980)*

er. But she felt chronically tired, because the frequent need to urinate and Matthew's kicks kept her awake through the night. Like many women, she began to look forward to delivery with a combination of apprehension and eagerness. Above all else, she was curious about the baby sharing her body. Was it a boy or a girl? Would its hair be red like hers or dark like Mark's? What color would its eyes be? The changes she had experienced so far seemed like only a prelude, and she waited restlessly for the day when she could meet her baby face to face.

· The Growing Baby

No one could pinpoint the precise moment at which Maryann's ovum and Mark's sperm combined to begin the long, intricate process of forming their son Matthew. As is usual, fertilization occurred in the upper part of the fallopian tube, and the first cell division took place within a day. As the fertilized egg floated gently down the tube, the cells continued to divide. However, the cells became smaller with each division, so the total cell unit stayed about the same size as the original fertilized ovum.

At the time the cluster of cells reached Maryann's uterus, it was still smaller than the head of a pin. Once nestled into the spongy uterine lining, the embryo, as it is called during the first two months, took on an elongated shape, rounded at one end. A sac (the amnion) enveloped it. As water and other small molecules crossed the amniotic membrane, the embryo was able to float freely in the absorbed fluid, cushioned from shocks and bumps. A primitive placenta began to form. Gradually it would take on the jobs of supplying the growing baby with food, water, and nutrients from the maternal bloodstream and of carrying waste back to Maryann's body for disposal. For Matthew, the placenta would serve as a combination of lungs, kidneys, and digestive system. For Maryann, it would act as a hormone gland, secreting estrogen and progesterone and regulating the schedule of physiological changes.

At the end of Matthew's first month in the womb, he was a quarter of an inch long—10,000 times his original size—and developing at amazing speed. His cells were differentiating into layers, tissues, and organs, grouping themselves according to the directions encoded in his genes. The neural tube, the beginning of the nervous system, was still open. There were gill-like arches that would develop into a mouth, lower jaw, and throat. Beneath them was a tiny U-shaped tube that would form his heart.

In the second month, the sculpting of Matthew's face began. Two tiny folds of tissue appeared on either side of his head; they would develop into ears. There was a tiny depression where his nose would be and a thickening that would become his tongue. His head, larger than the rest of his body, seemed to rest on his chest as if it were too heavy for him to hold up. His brain was developing rapidly, with the various sections, nerves, and membranes beginning to grow. Cartilage spread upward to enclose it, although Matthew's skull would not knit firmly together for almost a decade, when his brain finally stopped increasing in size. In medical terms, he became a fetus.

By the end of Matthew's third month, he was completely formed. His heart was beating rapidly. His face was modeled into a unique configuration of features. He could open his mouth, squint, purse his lips. The "buds" for his limbs had developed into arms and legs, and fingers and toes had been defined. Matthew began to exercise his muscles and to move freely within his fluid-filled capsule, but his mother could not yet detect any signs of his activity. Sexual organs appeared, as well as all other major internal organs.

Matthew grew rapidly in his fourth month, stretching to a length of more than 6 inches and a weight of 5 ounces. He began to drink some of the amniotic fluid, which his kidneys processed and passed as urine back into the amniotic sac. His heart could be heard through a special stethoscope. A temporary covering of hair grew on his eyebrows, palms, soles, and upper lip. His skeleton developed, with bone cells filling in and hardening the cartilage "molds."

In his fifth month, fine hair called lanugo, from the Latin word for down, covered his body. Most of this silky covering would rub off by birth. His eyes opened and closed. His ears were sensitive enough to detect sounds. Nails appeared on his fingers and toes, and the ridges on his palms and soles were fully formed. Matthew began testing his reflexes, grasping and sucking as well as kicking and moving. He still had plenty of room for somersaulting, but his mother now could feel his twists and turns and detect a daily pattern of activity and rest.

By the end of his sixth month, Matthew was 13 inches long and weighed more than 1½ pounds. Although his vital organs were quite developed, his lungs were not yet mature. If Matthew had been born at this time, he would have had only a fifty-fifty chance of surviving. A protective coating, called vernix, formed over the lanugo, clinging to the hairy parts and the creases of Matthew's body. His skin, once the color of old parchment, began to look more opaque, but it remained very wrinkled. If Maryann had been able to peek inside her womb, she might have thought that her son looked more like a tiny old man than the fat, pink babies that appear in diaper commercials.

In the last trimester, Matthew added inches and pounds to his frame. Much of the weight was deposited under his skin as fat. This fat layer would serve him well in providing necessary energy during birth and in maintaining his body temperature afterward. Gradually he took on a more "babylike" appearance, with pinkish skin and chubby limbs. In the last weeks in the womb, Matthew's lungs produced a crucial material that lines the small air sacs. This substance, surfactant, would assist him in breathing on his own. In preparation for breathing, he spent

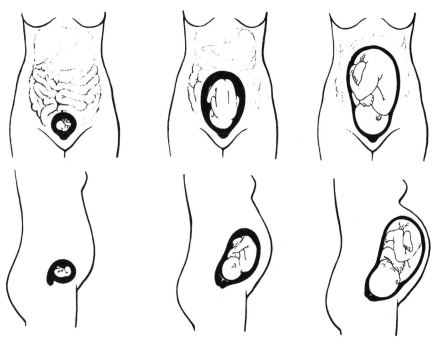

The relative size of the uterus and fetus at four, six and a half, and nine months of gestation *(from Reeder, Mastroianni, and Martin, Maternity Nursing, 14th ed. J. B. Lippincott, 1980)*

about half of his time making respirationlike movements. By the end of the eighth month, Matthew had adopted the typical head-down, or vertex, position in his mother's pear-shaped womb. In the ninth month, his head moved lower into her pelvis, like an egg settling into an egg cup. Rather than moving his entire body, he would just prod Maryann with an arm or a leg.

Nine months after Maryann's ovum was fertilized by Mark's sperm, the process of fetal development, growth, and maturation was complete. Two cells had grown to 6,000 billion cells. A heart had been working for months. A brain had begun to respond to stimuli. Arms and legs had grown just so much and no more. A face had formed with features that would distinguish Matthew Branley from all others. In the darkness of the womb, waiting to be born, lay a unique individual, ready to journey into the world.

• Becoming Parents

Not all of the changes of Maryann's pregnancy were physical. During the first trimester, she often felt that her feelings were changing more than her body was. Her initial joy at being pregnant faded during a long bout with morning sickness. Her moods would swing from tears to laughter in a matter of minutes. For a few weeks she withdrew into herself. Even though she wanted this child, she had days of depression and doubt. She worried about money, about medical complications, about the impact the baby would have on her marriage. Perhaps her greatest fear, however, was of the unknown. Sometimes she felt distressingly out of control of what was happening within and around her.

Mark also found that his wife's pregnancy triggered new feelings. Initially he was proud of siring a child, but that pride changed to a deep sense of responsibility. He began to reevaluate his job, salary, and plans for the future. His attitude toward Maryann changed. At times he found her more sexually attractive than ever, yet he was put off by her sudden mood shifts and uncertain about her concern for him as well as their baby. The pregnancy became more real and exciting for him when, in the fifth month, he was stroking Maryann's abdomen and felt the baby kick. It was as if he'd finally been introduced to his child, and he eagerly began making plans and thinking of names.

Ironically, both Maryann and Mark, on the verge of becoming parents, felt a great need for parenting themselves. Maryann turned to Mark for reassurance, affection, and support. Mark tried to be solicitous without being overprotective, yet had to contend with his own needs and doubts. They both found that the best way of handling their varied emotions was with openness. As they showed that they cared about each other's anxieties and expectations, they were able to understand each other's emotions and provide support and sympathy.

By the final trimester, Maryann and Mark had worked through their complicated feelings about having a child. They attended childbirth classes and set up the nursery together. While both worried about the difficulty of labor and delivery, they were caught up in another shared emotion—intense anticipation. In a sense, the nine months of waiting had been as crucial for them as for Matthew. During the time that he was preparing for life, they were preparing for the most demanding and rewarding roles of their lives—those of mother and father.

3 . Having a Healthy Baby

JOANNA PETERS ALWAYS WANTED to have children—but later rather than sooner. All through her twenties, she had other priorities. She wanted to finish graduate school, spend a year traveling, get her career off the ground, establish her professional reputation. After she married, she often was asked if she had children. "Not yet," she'd reply with a smile. But there always seemed to be a good reason for waiting just a little longer.

When Joanna turned 30, she and her husband talked more and more about having a baby. Maybe after they bought a bigger house. Or after they paid off the loan on the new car. Or after Bill's transfer to Houston came through. Their parents began to ask delicately phrased questions about whether there were any "problems" in having children. "None except finding the time," they said.

Then Joanna woke up on the morning of her thirty-fifth birthday. "I realized I had everything I'd always wanted, with one big exception—a baby. I panicked. I began to think that maybe I had waited too long and that now that I finally was ready, there would be problems. The next week I was in an obstetrician's office, asking if I was fit to become a mother."

The doctor was reassuring. Yes, Joanna was a bit beyond the ideal age for childbearing, and that meant an increased possibility of conceiving a baby with Down's syndrome (see page 35), a major genetic cause of mental retardation. However, a prenatal test could be performed to determine if her baby's genetic make-up was normal. But age was not Joanna's only risk factor. As her doctor explained, both her pack-a-day smoking and her chronic high blood pressure (hypertension) could be hazardous for an unborn baby. His advice was to start working to overcome these risks *before* she became pregnant.

In the next few months Joanna set out to get herself in shape for motherhood. She weaned herself from cigarettes. Through a combination of strict dietary control and exercise, she brought her blood pressure down within normal range. She told her friends that she'd never felt better in her life. And a few months later she succeeded in becoming pregnant.

Most mothers-to-be don't think about their health and habits until they're already pregnant. Joanna's approach to anticipating and overcoming risks is ideal. Preventive care is essential in guaranteeing a baby a healthy start in life. The months before your baby's birth are too important to take either your body or your baby for granted. As soon as you plan to become or discover you are pregnant, you should start taking very good care of yourself—for your sake and your baby's. In this chapter we'll describe the basics of good prenatal care and the risk factors that may require extra attention during pregnancy.

· Prenatal Care

Your baby is more dependent on you in the months before birth than it will be at any other time in its life. To assure your baby of the best possible care before birth, you should get a medical checkup as soon as you think you're pregnant. Your obstetrician will determine exactly how pregnant you are by figuring out when ovulation and fertilization probably occurred: two weeks after the first day of your last menstrual period. In order to estimate your delivery, or due, date, your physician will count 280 days, or 40 weeks, from the beginning of your last period. This is an accurate way of determining when a baby is due for about 85 percent of pregnant women. However, your cycles may be longer or shorter than 28 days, or they may be quite irregular. It often takes several months to reestablish regular cycles after discontinuing oral contraceptives, so if you recently stopped taking the pill, your estimated delivery date may be more of an approximation than a precise target date. Your doctor may try to get a better idea of your baby's age by other methods, such as a sonogram (ultrasonic examination) in the first half of pregnancy (see page 41). Particularly in high-risk pregnancies, accurate dating of your pregnancy can be critically important. If your baby should require treatment before birth or shows signs of distress in the womb, your obstetrician will need to know its exact gestational age to aid in deciding on a form of treatment or on an early delivery.

Your doctor also will check your weight and blood pressure; these measurements will serve as the basis for assessing changes during pregnancy. You will be given a complete physical, including a pelvic or vaginal exam. At subsequent visits, your doctor will evaluate your uterus and baby by palpating your abdomen. Your "fundal height"—the distance between your pubic bone and the top of your uterus, or fundus—will be checked. Normally fundal height increases steadily until the last month or so, when the baby settles into the pelvis and there is a slight decrease. If your measurements don't follow the usual pattern, your baby may be younger than its estimated age or may have impaired growth.

Your obstetrician will get considerable information about your health from laboratory tests of your blood and urine. A count of your red blood cells will indicate if you have too few of these crucial oxygen-carrying cells; this is a sign of anemia (see page 114). A high number of white blood cells may indicate infection. Your physician also will check your blood type to see if there may be any potential incompatibility problems, such as Rh sensitization. Another blood test, required by law, indicates whether you have a venereal disease. If you have not been vaccinated against rubella (German measles), your doctor will check to see if you had acquired natural immunity to this virus prior to pregnancy. If not, you should be vaccinated *after* your pregnancy has ended.

Analysis of a sample of your first urine of the day will reveal the presence of any bacteria. Women with bacteria in their urine—even without any symptoms of a urinary tract infection—are more likely to develop a serious urine infection before delivery. An unusually large amount of protein in your urine (a condition called proteinuria) can indicate a kidney problem. The amount of glucose (sugar) in your urine reflects how well you are metabolizing foods; a high glucose level means increased risk of developing a condition similar to diabetes during pregnancy.

If your pregnancy is uncomplicated, you will return to your doctor's office approximately once a month during the first and second trimesters, at two- or three-week intervals during your seventh and eighth months, and weekly during your ninth month. Most of these visits will be much briefer than your initial exam. Your doctor will record your weight gain to make sure your baby is growing as it should, measure fundal height, and palpate your abdomen. He or she will check your blood pressure carefully and perform urine, blood, or other tests if there are any suspected problems.

Each prenatal visit is a chance for you, as well as your obstetrician, to ask questions and gather information. The relationship the two of you develop may be different from other interactions you've had with physicians. Rather than being the passive, ill recipient of treatment, you can be an involved participant, working with your doctor to help your baby in every possible way. That is why it is critical that you choose an obstetrician whom you can talk with easily and whom you trust. Once you make the choice, you should rely on your doctor's judgment and understanding of what is best for your baby.

Since you may find it difficult to remember all the questions that come up between visits, try to keep a list and take it with you on your next visit. Don't worry that your concerns may seem trivial or take up too much of your doctor's time. Any problem or fear that is troubling you is worth mentioning to your obstetrician.

· Taking Care of Yourself

Pregnancy is a unique physiological experience during which many basic functions do not go on as usual. Your appearance, metabolism, respiration, circulation, and digestion all undergo changes. For your baby's sake and your own comfort, you may want to make some other changes—in your habits, your schedule, and your self-expectations.

Nutrition

What you eat during pregnancy has a profound effect on your well-being and on your baby's growth and development. Poor nutrition during pregnancy increases the risk of complications, stillbirths, and birth defects. Whenever the diets of malnourished pregnant women have been improved, they have had fewer problems before delivery and their babies have encountered fewer difficulties after birth.

Your baby's weight at birth will be affected by the amount of weight you gain during pregnancy. Infants with very low birth weights are at much greater risk of mental retardation and developmental problems than babies who weigh just a pound or two more.

In a society as waistline-conscious as ours, gaining weight can seem like a social sin. Pregnancy, however, is no time for dieting. It is far more important to provide your growing baby with the nutrients it needs than to worry about fitting into the clothes you once wore. The National Academy of Sciences and the National Research Council's Committee on Maternal Nutrition recommend a minimum weight gain of 24 to 27 pounds during pregnancy. Underweight women should gain at least 30 pounds to make sure their babies' nutritional needs are met.

The ideal pattern for weight gain is to add pounds slowly. During the first trimester you should gain a total of 2 to 4 pounds. In the second and third trimesters, you should gain a little less than a pound a week for a total of about 22 to 24 pounds. At delivery, your baby will account for about 7½ pounds of your increased weight. The placenta will weigh 1½ pounds; your uterus, 2 pounds; your breasts, 4 pounds. Increased blood volume and body fluids add another 8½ pounds. If you gain more weight than is advised early in pregnancy, do *not* try to make up for it by dieting later. Such restrictions can harm your baby and interfere with your ability to maintain an adequate energy reserve for yourself. Report any sudden, substantive weight gain (for example, five pounds in a single week) to your doctor; it could mean that you are retaining excessive fluids or having blood pressure or kidney problems.

The quality of the foods you eat while pregnant is as important as the quantity of weight you gain. During pregnancy you will be synthesizing complex new tissues at a faster rate than at any other time of your life, so protein is critical. Your daily diet should also include foods from the four other basic food groups: milk and milk products, grain products, vitamin C–rich fruits and vegetables, leafy green vegetables and other produce. Your doctor may recommend an iron supplement. (See Appendix A for a sample daily diet.)

Exercise

The time when a pregnant woman was "confined" to her bed to wait for her baby's arrival is long past. You will be encouraged to exercise throughout your pregnancy if no obvious problems arise. If you were athletic before pregnancy, you can continue your favorite sports, although you may have to modify your style. Your center of gravity will change along with your body's bulk, so you may find walking more comfortable than running and doubles tennis much easier than singles. Try to avoid pushing yourself to the point of exhaustion or overheating. Your body will give you signals as to how much exercise is too much. Many exercise studios now offer special classes for mothers-to-be that provide an opportunity for you to stay fit and also to talk with other women expecting babies.

Sex

Many women report some changes in their sexual attitudes during pregnancy. Often they become less interested in sex in the first trimester but much more so in the second trimester. Most couples can continue to have intercourse until the membranes of the amniotic sac rupture and/or labor begins. You should abstain, however, if you begin to bleed from your vagina or if you are at high risk of preterm labor and delivery. A research team that reviewed the medical records of several thousand pregnant women in the 1960s did find a correlation between sex in the last month of pregnancy and neonatal infection, but its findings have been disputed. Some obstetricians recommend the use of condoms during intercourse.

Travel

You can continue to drive as long as you can fit behind the wheel comfortably. Short car trips—as driver or passenger—usually are no problem. However, sitting in one place for too long a time can interfere with the flow of blood to your legs and feet. Schedule rest stops every two hours or so, and get up and walk around. Moving your feet frequently while sitting also can help prevent problems.

You can travel by plane as long as you are flying in a pressurized commercial aircraft. If you are in your last trimester, some airlines may require a letter from your doctor saying that it is all right for you to travel. Your doctor may advise you not to fly in your final month because of concern about an airborne delivery. If your pregnancy is complicated, you may want to reconsider any trips that may cause extra strain or that may take you away from available perinatal services.

Work

Most pregnant women can work until the final days of pregnancy, depending on the nature of their jobs. Very strenuous occupations or jobs that require long hours on your feet may cause too much physical strain, and you may be advised to cut back your hours. If you develop problems in pregnancy, your obstetrician may advise you to stop working in order to avoid unnecessary physical and emotional demands. The same cautions apply to housework and domestic chores.

Stress

Psychological problems, like physical ones, can make any pregnancy more difficult. A woman alone, or carrying an unwanted child, or isolated from friends and family is much more vulnerable. Situational stresses, such as worry about a job or money, the loss of a loved one, or a divorce, add to the emotional demands of pregnancy. Because the mind and body are interdependent, it often is impossible to say which comes first—the emotional stress or the medical complication. If you are encountering emotional difficulties, try to find someone to talk to— your doctor, a nurse, a social worker, a friend. Such support can ease your worries and help you cope, indirectly helping your baby as well.

Physical Discomforts

As your body changes and your baby grows, you may experience symptoms ranging from trivial to troublesome. It may help to know that many such discomforts are common and temporary. The chart that follows lists the most frequent complaints of pregnant women along with their causes, suggestions for prevention, and recommended treatments.

COMMON DISCOMFORTS AND WHAT TO DO ABOUT THEM

Nausea and indigestion; shortness of breath

Concentrate on good posture, pulling in your abdominal muscles and tilting your pelvis, to give the stomach and lungs more room. Try sleeping on extra pillows to elevate your head and chest. Eat small meals every two to three hours rather than three larger meals. Avoid liquids with meals, acid- or gas-producing foods, and an empty stomach.

Pelvic pressure; thigh-hip pain; heaviness in legs; backache

Practice good posture while sitting, standing, and lifting. Using your abdominal muscles, try to lift the baby up off the big blood vessels in the pelvis and nerves that might be pinched. Relieve strain on your back with ample rest periods. Try pillow support under your top leg and arms and uterus to relieve the pull on your back.

Stretch marks

May be reduced by good posture to reduce pressure and stretching of the abdomen.

Swelling of the feet; varicose veins

Good posture and ample rest will help. You can improve circulation by raising your legs to drain fluid from them. Lie on the bed or floor with a pillow under your hips. Raise your legs up on the wall with knees bent and slowly make circles with your feet to the right and left. Point your heel rather than your toe. If you wear elastic support hose, drain your legs this way *before* putting on your stockings. Change body position often; wear sensible shoes and clothing that does not bind.

Swelling of the hands

Slight swelling of the fingers is common. Drink six to eight glasses of water daily and maintain a good diet, high in protein. Restrict salt only if instructed by doctor.

Leg cramps

These are common in the last three months because of the drain of calcium from your system for the baby's bone growth and decreased circulation as a result of the pressure of the growing baby. Adequate calcium in the diet—from dairy products, dark green vegetables, or calcium lactate (only if prescribed by your doctor)—is essential. Practice good posture. Straighten cramped muscles by standing up. Try warm baths, loose covers over your feet, pillows under your legs.

Constipation

Moderate exercise will help. Maintain intake of roughage in diet (fruits, whole grains, bran, raw vegetables). Increase fluids. Establish regular bowel habits; respond quickly to the urge to eliminate. Try relaxation and deep breathing during elimination to relax the anal sphincter. Use stool softeners only if prescribed.

Hemorrhoids (rectal varicosities)

Avoid constipation. Good posture will help to prevent pooling of blood in the rectal area. Try elevation of hips and extremities. Try soaking in a warm tub or applying witch hazel or Tucks to affected area.

Pelvic cramps during intercourse

Choose positions in which you can bend your knees. Ask your partner to massage your lower abdomen gently. Penetration should be shallow.

Fatigue/insomnia

Try deep breathing for relaxation and good pillow support for comfort. Sleep on your side with pillows under your top leg and arm and under your uterus. Or try a semisitting position, with pillows under your back, knees, and arms. Keep your feet up as much as possible during the day.

Dizziness

Get up slowly, moving your arms and legs to increase blood flow. Roll over onto your side and push yourself up with your hands to avoid back strain.

Feeling of warmth; heavy bodily secretions; oily hair

These are all caused by hormonal changes and increased metabolism. Wear cool, loose, comfortable clothing. You may feel more comfortable if you bathe and wash your hair more frequently.

· Recognizing the Risks

The course of a pregnancy does not always run smoothly. The process of forming a new life is complex, and it may be more remarkable that so many pregnancies are uncomplicated than that problems can and do arise.

Obstetricians can identify at least half of the women who will eventually develop problems during pregnancy or delivery at the first prenatal visit and another 25 percent before labor begins. Such early awareness of a potential problem can prevent its occurrence or minimize its effects. An estimated 25 percent of the diseases, defects, and deaths that occur in the perinatal period could be prevented if treatment began early enough in pregnancy.

As they've learned how critical the period before birth is, obstetricians have begun to screen pregnant women for possible risk factors. As you review the details of your family, medical, and reproductive history, you may think that your doctor is looking for trouble. In a sense, that's right. But more precisely, your doctor wants to know about the *potential* for danger in order to safeguard you and your baby from possible hazards.

One or two of every ten pregnant women is classified as being at risk during the first prenatal visit. Finding out that you are a high-risk mother may sound more alarming than it really is. This categorization does not mean that you are destined to have problems during pregnancy or that your baby's life is in jeopardy. Rather, it is a signal to your doctor that you may need extra attention and care to ensure a successful pregnancy and a healthy baby.

Keep in mind that not all risk factors are equally serious. Being overweight may have a minimal effect on your pregnancy. If you also have high blood pressure, there's an additional risk. Again, if your blood pressure is elevated only slightly above normal, you are much less likely to encounter problems than if you have severe hypertension and associated kidney problems.

The following discussion of risk factors should give you a better idea of whether you'll need to take special precautions during pregnancy.

Age

Pregnancy is possible from menarche, the beginning of menstruation, until menopause. In the United States, the mean age for menarche is 12.3 years, but much younger girls have conceived and delivered babies. The youngest verified mother was a 5-year-old Peruvian girl. The prime time for having babies, according to data correlating maternal age with perinatal deaths, is between the ages of 25 and 29. The incidence of fetal loss is almost as low in women between the ages of 20 and 24 and between 30 and 34. Those who are considerably younger or older are statistically at greater risk of losing their babies before or shortly after birth.

Teenage mothers are at increased risk for a variety of reasons, including physiological and psychological immaturity. Pregnant adolescents are more likely to deliver prematurely, to have difficult labors, and to have babies less likely to survive. However, such complications may not be inevitable. At one perinatal center a team of physicians, social workers, dieticians, and teachers worked closely with a group of teenage mothers, educating them and providing good prenatal care. The girls had fewer preterm births, shorter and less complicated deliveries, and a perinatal mortality rate lower than the national average for mothers of all ages.

The "mature" or older mother usually has quite different concerns. According to national statistics, women between the ages of 35 and 39 deliver some 225,000 babies a year, about 7 percent of all births. This number and percentage are expected to increase as more women who have postponed childbearing conceive in their mid or late thirties. For most of these women, age is not a serious risk factor—particularly if they have no chronic medical problems, receive good prenatal care, and are in good physical condition. The risks do increase for women over 40, particularly if they are "primigravidas," or first-time mothers. In one study of women between the ages of 40 and 54, there was a higher-than-usual incidence of infants with low birth weights, and the newborn mortality rate was 10 percent, much higher than the average for women of all ages. The most common complication among these women was hypertension.

Older mothers also are more likely to have other medical conditions associated with increasing age, such as atherosclerosis (narrowing of the arteries). Often related to hypertension, this problem can affect the blood flow to the uterus and the growing baby. The incidence of abnormalities of the reproductive organs increases with age, but these problems usually are a greater threat to fertility than to a successful pregnancy. About 20 percent of women over 35 have fibroid tumors (myomas), benign growths in the uterus that may increase the risk of miscarriage, preterm birth, or difficult labor. Some obstetricians have reported that older mothers have longer and more complicated labors, with slower dilation of the cervix (because the uterine muscles lose their tone with time), and with more bleeding during delivery. Older women have more cesarean (abdominal) deliveries, although the reasons do not seem to be related to age but to specific medical problems and a very cautious obstetrical approach.

Every woman over 35 faces a greater risk of having a baby with Down's syndrome, a devastating chromosomal defect that causes mental retardation and other abnormalities (see Chapter 4). A genetics counselor can explain the risks and benefits of amniocentesis, a test that can detect this problem in the first half of a pregnancy.

Weight

Your baby's weight depends to a great extent on the amount of time it spends in your womb and on how much weight you gain during pregnancy. Your prepregnancy weight is important in evaluating potential risks to you and your baby.

If you weighed 10 percent *less* than the ideal weight for your height prior to conception, you have an increased chance of preterm labor and of delivering a lighter, shorter baby than usual. You may be able to overcome this risk by gaining more than the typical recommended amount of weight. A gain of about 30 pounds can reduce the risk of having a low-birth-weight or preterm infant.

If you weighed 10 percent *more* than you ideally should, you face a greater risk of developing blood pressure problems or a condition resembling diabetes during pregnancy. That doesn't mean you should diet, but you should monitor what you eat, for problems caused by poor nutrition can be extremely serious for your baby. Most overweight women are examined more often during pregnancy so an obstetrician or a nutrition expert can keep tabs on their diet and general well-being. Some studies suggest that overweight women have longer labors, with more delays and complications. A cesarean delivery is not more likely, but if it should be necessary—as with any surgery for overweight women—the extra pounds can increase the likelihood of problems related to anesthesia, bleeding, infection, and healing.

Chronic Illness

Your baby's health will reflect your own well-being, and any illness that affects your health can affect your baby. It is impossible to generalize about the impact that pregnancy can have on a medical problem or that a chronic illness can have on pregnancy. The chapters in Part 2,

"Problems Along the Way," discuss the possible risks and available treatments for the most common medical complications of pregnancy, including hypertension, heart disorders, respiratory ailments, digestive complaints, blood abnormalities, diabetes, kidney disease, thyroid disorders, infections, neurological problems, and gynecologic abnormalities.

Reproductive History

Your doctor will ask detailed questions about any previous pregnancies, miscarriages, and abortions because every pregnancy—regardless of its outcome—may have some impact on subsequent ones. Simply being a first-time mother is significant because of the unknowns of a first pregnancy and the typically longer course of labor and delivery. Two or more induced abortions, particularly in the second trimester, may increase the probability of problems if the procedures caused damage to the cervix or the uterine wall. A series of three or more miscarriages may be chance occurrences or a sign of an underlying problem.

If you delivered any of your children early, you face a 25 percent chance of another preterm birth. If your children were small or large for their gestational age, their size may reflect a medical problem that could affect your next baby. If you had a baby that was stillborn or died within a month of birth, your doctor will want to know as many specifics as possible about your experience to ensure that this sad event does not recur. If any of your children have congenital defects, your obstetrician may refer you to a genetics counselor. You also should report any complications you encountered during a previous delivery. If you had a cesarean delivery your obstetrician will want to know the reasons and the type of incision used in delivering the baby through your abdomen (see Chapter 20). This information may determine whether you can attempt a vaginal delivery this time.

Your obstetrician will ask if you've had problems getting pregnant. If you had been trying to conceive for more than a year without success, you may need special attention during pregnancy, depending on the suspected cause of your difficulty. Certain gynecologic disorders, for example, may increase the risks of miscarriage. Neither you nor your doctor will want to risk losing a baby that you've tried so long to conceive.

If you became pregnant with an intrauterine device (IUD) in place, your obstetrician may remove it to eliminate any risk of infection. You should tell your doctor if you continued to take birth control pills after conceiving; prolonged use of oral contraceptives after conception slightly increases the risk of heart and limb malformations.

If you became pregnant within three months of your last delivery, you may not have had time to recover from the enormous physiological upheaval of pregnancy and delivery. Women who have had six or more deliveries—"grand multiparas"—are at increased risk, particularly of bleeding excessively during their next delivery.

Problems in Your Current Pregnancy

Many of the normal changes of pregnancy—shortness of breath, palpitations of the heart, increased urination—might seem decidedly abnormal at any other time of your life. While these are not a cause for alarm, there are other symptoms that actually may be signals of increasing danger to you or your baby. You should notify your doctor immediately if you develop any of the following problems:

• *Vaginal bleeding.* Approximately 20 to 25 percent of pregnant women spot or bleed lightly in the first months of pregnancy, particularly on the days when menstruation might normally have occurred. Bleeding in the first half of pregnancy also can be a sign of impending miscarriage. In the second and third trimester, it may indicate that the placenta is covering the opening of the uterus (a condition called placenta previa) or that the placenta is separating from the uterine wall before delivery (a placental abruption).

• *Abdominal pain.* Early in pregnancy, cramplike pain may be a sign of miscarriage. In the second half of pregnancy, such pain may indicate preterm labor or placental abruption.

• *Nausea and vomiting.* An estimated 40 percent of all pregnant women have some digestive discomfort in the first trimester. If nausea and vomiting are extremely severe or persistent, you may require medical treatment (Chapter 15).

• *Unusual thirst.* This is a classic sign of diabetes. Your doctor may want you to undergo tests for gestational diabetes (see Chapter 13).

• *Chills or fever.* These symptoms of infectious disease may signal the need for prompt medical treatment.

• *Swelling of your face or fingers.* It's not unusual for your feet and ankles to become swollen during pregnancy. However, if your face and hands begin to swell, you may be developing blood pressure or kidney problems (see chapters 11 and 14).

• *Severe or continuous headaches.* You may have occasional headaches during pregnancy—just as at any other time—but you should report any persistent or unusually severe headaches. They could be another sign of blood pressure problems (see Chapter 11).

• *Dimness or blurring of vision.* This symptom also can indicate that your blood pressure is rising and that you need immediate treatment.

• *Fluid leaking from your vagina.* A sudden gush of fluid early in pregnancy may indicate a miscarriage. Later in pregnancy, it may mean that the membranes of your amniotic sac have ruptured and that labor may begin prematurely (see Chapter 9).

4 . Genetic Risks: Yesterdays and Tomorrows

THE WAITING ROOM is filled with couples, mostly in their twenties and thirties. Some hold hands; some pace; some flip through magazines, ignoring the words and glancing at the photographs. Other patients in other offices might act in much the same way, but this group is unusual. These men and women, all in the prime of their lives, have not come for help because of worry about their own well-being. What concerns them is not the present but the past and the future: the genetic legacy they've received from their parents and the genetic risks they might pass on to their unborn children.

Like these couples at a genetic counseling center, all parents would like to peer into the future for assurance that their babies will be perfect in every way. There are no crystal balls available, but medical genetics, a relative newcomer among clinical specialties, has made great progress in identifying those parents at highest risk of having a child with a genetic disorder and in developing prenatal tests for detecting such problems early in pregnancy. In this chapter we'll describe the basic mechanisms of heredity, the most common genetic ailments, and the new options for parents.

· Genes and Chromosomes

The basic units of heredity that link past, present, and future are genes, tiny molecules of DNA—the fundamental "stuff" of life—that determine how you develop. Every cell in your body has a nucleus containing thousands of genes, arranged on twenty-three pairs of rodlike structures called chromosomes. One pair, the sex chromosome, determines the sex of an individual. A woman has two X chromosomes in every cell nucleus; a man has an X and a Y. The other twenty-two pairs of chromosomes, which govern all other aspects of development, are called autosomes. The autosomes in these pairs are usually identical in size and shape.

Genes also occur in pairs, with each gene occupying a specific location, or locus, on a particular chromosome. The two genes that occupy precise locations on a pair of chromosomes are called alleles. You have two alleles for every genetic trait.

Not all genes have equal influence. Some are "dominant" and exert their influence—or in medical terms, "express themselves"—even if carried on only one of a pair of chromosomes. As the drawings on pages 31–33 illustrate, every child conceived by a father carrying a single faulty dominant gene and a normal mother has a 50 percent chance of inheriting the abnormal trait. The less-influential "recessive" genes are "masked" by dominant genes; they express themselves only if a child inherits two of the same recessive genes. If both parents carry the same faulty recessive gene, each child they conceive faces a 25 percent risk of inheriting a "double dose" of the defect (a faulty gene

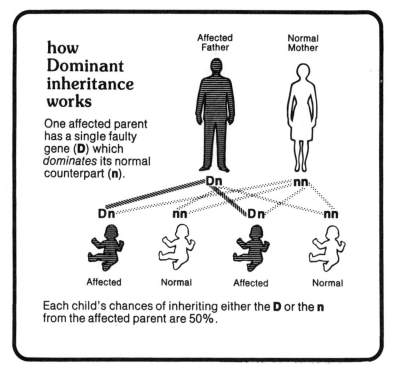

how **Dominant inheritance works**

One affected parent has a single faulty gene (**D**) which *dominates* its normal counterpart (**n**).

Affected Father

Normal Mother

Dn   **nn**

Dn   **nn**   **Dn**   **nn**

Affected   Normal   Affected   Normal

Each child's chances of inheriting either the **D** or the **n** from the affected parent are 50%.

(March of Dimes Birth Defects Foundation)

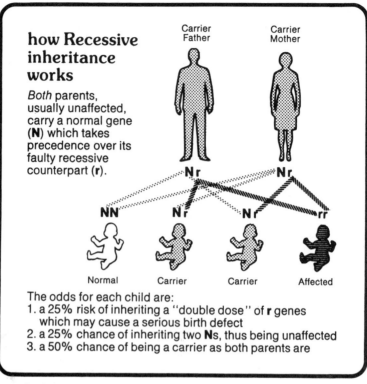

how Recessive inheritance works

Both parents, usually unaffected, carry a normal gene **(N)** which takes precedence over its faulty recessive counterpart (**r**).

Carrier Father

Carrier Mother

N r   **N r**

NN   **N r**   **N r**   **rr**

Normal   Carrier   Carrier   Affected

The odds for each child are:
1. a 25% risk of inheriting a "double dose" of **r** genes which may cause a serious birth defect
2. a 25% chance of inheriting two **N**s, thus being unaffected
3. a 50% chance of being a carrier as both parents are

(March of Dimes Birth Defects Foundation)

from each parent), a 25 percent chance of inheriting two normal genes and not being affected, and a 50 percent chance for inheriting an abnormal gene from only one parent and becoming a carrier for the defect. A recessive gene on the X chromosome may express itself only in men; this is called an X-linked trait. The odds for each male child of a woman with a defective gene on her X chromosome are 50 percent for inheriting the faulty X and the disorder and 50 percent for inheriting the normal X. For each female child, the odds are 50 percent for inheriting one faulty X and becoming a carrier like her mother and 50 percent for inheriting the normal X and no defective gene.

Your genes and chromosomes affect every conceivable aspect of your appearance, well-being, likelihood of developing certain illnesses, even your longevity and behavior. Medical genetics—the study of heredity—is one of the most complex of medical sciences, as well as one of the most sophisticated. Yet a great deal about how genes affect our lives is still unknown. The basic information in this chapter cannot answer all your questions about the genes you inherited from your parents and those you may pass on to your children. However, it may make you more aware of the profound influence genes have on your present and on your children's future.

· Genetic Errors: What Can Go Wrong

The blueprints for life encoded in our genes are so detailed and intricate that it's not surprising that occasional mistakes occur. What *is* surprising is that more mistakes don't occur more often. Of every one hundred newborns, only two to four have any sort of genetic defect, yet all parents worry about the possibility of a genetic flaw. It's true that, in a sense, each of us is a carrier of a genetic problem. Every individual has an estimated four to eight defective genes, but the chances that they will affect your child are slight. Almost always these genes are recessive and do not express themselves. The likelihood of your child inheriting a faulty recessive gene from you and the same abnormal gene from your spouse is remote—unless you marry someone with a genetic makeup very similar to your own, such as a first cousin.

Geneticists classify hereditary problems according to the way in

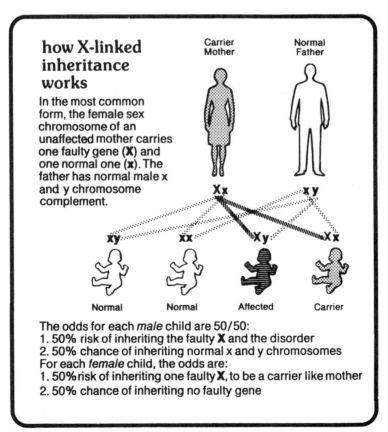

how X-linked inheritance works

In the most common form, the female sex chromosome of an unaffected mother carries one faulty gene (**X**) and one normal one (**x**). The father has normal male x and y chromosome complement.

Carrier Mother

Normal Father

Xx   **xy**

xy   **xx**   **Xy**   **Xx**

Normal   Normal   Affected   Carrier

The odds for each *male* child are 50/50:
1. 50% risk of inheriting the faulty **X** and the disorder
2. 50% chance of inheriting normal x and y chromosomes
For each *female* child, the odds are:
1. 50% risk of inheriting one faulty **X**, to be a carrier like mother
2. 50% chance of inheriting no faulty gene

(March of Dimes Birth Defects Foundation)

which they originate. The causes can involve a single gene: defective autosomal dominant genes (carried by a dominant gene on one of the autosomes), defective autosomal recessive genes (carried by a recessive gene on two of the chromosomes), or sex-linked abnormalities (carried by an X chromosome). Or they can be chromosomal defects (abnormalities of any of the forty-six chromosomes), mutations (spontaneous changes in genes), or multifactorial problems.

Single-Gene Defects

A child of a parent with an abnormal dominant gene has a 50 percent likelihood of inheriting it. The most common of these defects are minor, such as polydactyly (the growth of an extra finger or toe). However, some uncommon autosomal dominant problems can be fatal—and may not be diagnosed for decades after birth. Huntington's chorea, for example, is a degenerative disease usually not diagnosed until mid life. There is no way to detect this inherited problem until symptoms develop, no treatment for the progressive loss of motor and mental skills, and no way to forestall inevitable death.

The effects of a dominant abnormal gene vary considerably from individual to individual, even from parent to child. Not everyone who inherits the defective gene for a disorder will develop it· this is a phenomenon called incomplete penetrance. A defective dominant gene that does express itself also can cause a spectrum of effects, ranging from minor symptoms in one person to multiple defects in another.

Far more common are autosomal recessive disorders. In American whites, the most common of these problems is cystic fibrosis, a debilitating disease of the sweat and mucous glands. In American blacks, the most frequent problem of this type is sickle-cell anemia (page 114). A "carrier," a person with the defective recessive gene, may never develop any symptoms, though the gene may be transmitted to his or her children. Blood tests can identify carriers of some of the most serious of these diseases, including beta-thalassemia (a blood disorder found in families of Mediterranean origin), Tay-Sachs (a deadly metabolic illness that strikes Jews of Eastern European background), and sickle-cell anemia.

Only women are carriers of X-linked problems, and only their sons are at risk. A boy faces a fifty-fifty chance of inheriting a defective gene on his mother's sex chromosome. A daughter also may inherit the gene and become a carrier, but she will not develop the symptoms because of the matching healthy gene on her other X chromosome. The most common X-linked problems are hemophilia, the "bleeder's disease," and Duchenne's muscular dystrophy, an impairment of muscle tissue.

Chromosomal Defects

Since a chromosomal flaw involves a much larger part of the genetic material than a single-gene defect, it has a much more devastating effect. While an abnormal gene might cause a problem similar to the misspelling of a word in this book, a chromosomal error could be compared to leaving out an entire chapter or putting it in the wrong sequence. Chromosomal defects occur much less frequently than single-gene flaws—in an estimated 1 of every 200 conceptions. Very often they result in miscarriages (see Chapter 7).

Sometimes one complete extra chromosome is added to the normal 46 in every cell in the body; this is called a trisomy. The best-known trisomy is Down's syndrome (once called mongolism). One of every 700 conceptions results in a fetus with Down's syndrome. Some do not survive until delivery; those who do are born with a cluster of physical and intellectual defects. They tend to be short and small, with stubby fingers and toes and flabby arms and legs. Their faces are flat, with a low bridge over the nose and a vaguely Oriental slant to their eyes. These babies always have some degree of mental retardation, although it can range from moderate to severe. Most can learn to walk, dress themselves, say some words, and perform simple tasks. Forty to 60 percent have heart defects; all face an increased risk of leukemia. About 25 percent do not survive their first year, and another 25 percent die by age 8 or 10.

For reasons that are not clearly understood, the incidence of chromosomal errors increases with age. Throughout her twenties, a woman's chance of having a baby with Down's syndrome is quite low—approximately 1 in 1,500. At age 30 the risk is 1 in 1,000; at 40; it's 1 in 100; at 45, 1 in 30.

Parents with defects in their own chromosomes also are more likely to have children with a similar problem. In one example of such a disorder, a parent may have a "translocation" defect, in which part or all of a particular chromosome is exchanged with another one. This disorder can result in a defective fetus and an early miscarriage. About 7,000 babies are born with translocation defects annually. One of the more frequent is a hereditary form of Down's syndrome.

Some individuals have both normal and abnormal sex chromosomes that form a "mosaic" of genetic material in their cells. Within some of the nuclei, there may be a normal XX or XY pair of chromosomes, while in others there will be an XXY or XYY grouping. The impact of this problem can range from severe malformations and retardation to effects so slight that the defect may never be noticed.

One of every 400 boys is born with an extra X chromosome, a problem known as Klinefelter's syndrome. The XXY configuration is the single most common cause of infertility in adult males, and it also increases the possibility of mental retardation. The only chromosomal disorder in which an individual can survive with fewer than forty-six chromosomes is Turner's syndrome. A person with this abnormality has only one sex chromosome, an X, in every cell. The typical consequences include a webbed neck, short stature, infantile development of female sex organs in maturity, and malformations of the eyelids, ears, and forearms.

Mutations

Some defects are the result of a spontaneous change in the makeup of a gene. Most such "mutations" occur without any known reason, although exposure to high levels of radiation—such as those produced by the atomic bomb explosions over Japan in World War II—is clearly linked to mutations and birth defects. Other environmental agents also may increase the risk of mutations, but very little is known about which ones may affect gene replication.

Multifactorial Defects

Many genetic disorders are the result of a combination of causes, including both familial inheritance and environmental factors. There is no clear pattern to why and when these multifactorial defects occur. The most common ones affect the neural tube, the precursor of the backbone, spinal cord, and brain in the embryo. If the top end of this cylindrical structure does not close in the first month of pregnancy, the unborn baby will not develop a normal brain; this condition, called anencephaly, is always fatal. If there is a flaw in the formation of the lower part of the tube, the spinal cord and nerves will remain outside the body. Surgery after birth can close this opening, but usually a baby with this disorder, known as spina bifida, remains paralyzed from the waist down and is incapable of acquiring bladder or bowel control. Many babies with spina bifida also develop hydrocephalus, an accumulation of fluid within the skull, and may be mentally retarded. The damage is less severe in a "closed" neural tube defect. For reasons we do not know, the incidence of neural tube defects varies in different countries and regions. They occur most frequently in Ireland; in the U.S. the incidence is higher in the Northeast than in southern California. In most cases, the chance that parents who've had one child with a neural tube defect will have another affected baby is 1 to 5 percent. However, a British research team has found a link between neural tube defects and nutritional deficiencies. In one study, women who had one baby with this type of defect seemed less likely to have another affected child if given multivitamin supplements before and during pregnancy.

· Prenatal Diagnosis

In the past two decades, scientists have developed ways of studying samples of fetal cells and detecting more than one hundred genetic disorders. The ability to learn about such problems early in pregnancy has changed many would-be parents' outlook on having children." In one study of the impact of genetic counseling services, more couples chose to conceive a child *after* learning about the risks than decided against becoming parents. A major reason was the availability of prenatal tests, including:

• *Amniocentesis*, a method of analyzing fetal cells for chromosomal defects, including Down's syndrome. It is recommended for all women over 35 because of the increased risk of chromosomal disorders, for mothers who have already borne children with genetic and chromosomal abnormalities, for women who may be carriers of X-linked disorders (to determine if the fetus is male and, therefore, at risk), and for couples who both carry a recessive trait for a disease. The test is described on page 44.

• *Ultrasound*, a technique for detecting such structural defects as hydrocephalus, spina bifida, and anencephaly (see page 41).

• *Fetoscopy*, a delicate procedure for peering within the womb and obtaining blood or skin samples for diagnosis of rare familial disorders (see page 47).

• *Alpha Fetal Protein Levels*, a measurement of a protein manufactured mainly in the liver of a fetus and released into the amniotic fluid when the fetus urinates. Normally alpha fetal protein (AFP) reaches its peak level in the fetus in the fourteenth week of pregnancy and then slowly decreases. The amount of AFP in the mother's blood typically increases until the middle of the third trimester. If a fetus has an open neural tube defect, such as spina bifida or anencephaly, the level of AFP in the amniotic fluid and in the mother's blood will be much higher. By measuring the AFP level in a woman's bloodstream at a given point in pregnancy, the obstetrician can detect a possible neural tube defect.

This testing, widespread in England but not in the U.S., does not yield clear-cut results. The AFP level sometimes is higher if the woman is carrying twins or if she is a week or two more pregnant than had been estimated. A second blood test is generally performed to rule out deceptive or false-positive results. If the AFP level is still significantly higher than normal, an ultrasonic scan may determine if there are twins or triplets in the womb or if there is an obvious neural tube defect, such as anencephaly. If the ultrasound still does not yield conclusive results, the obstetrician performs an amniocentesis to sample the amniotic fluid for AFP.

· Parents at Risk

Some genetic defects occur randomly. Much more often there is a pattern to their occurrence. As geneticists have learned more about the way one generation transmits a defect to another, they've been able to counsel parents about the potential risks to their unborn children. Today there is a network of genetic counseling centers across the country, staffed by physicians or specially trained "genetic associates" and equipped with computerized information-retrieval systems that provide immediate access to the facts and statistics about certain problems.

Genetic counseling is recommended for certain groups of parents most likely to have children with defects, including:

• women over age 35
• parents of a child with a single-gene abnormality, a neural tube defect, or another form of physical or mental impairment
• women who've had three or more miscarriages
• couples with chromosomal abnormalities
• women who may be carriers of X-linked disorders
• couples whose family members have a high incidence of certain diseases or unusually frequent cases of cancer or heart disease
• couples whose ethnic or racial backgrounds increase the likelihood of a particular problem, such as sickle-cell anemia or Tay-Sachs disease.

There is a new group of mothers at risk: the first generation of young women successfully treated for phenylketonuria (PKU). This is a hereditary metabolic disorder caused by lack of an enzyme that metabolizes the compound phenylalanine, which can build up in body fluids and cause mental retardation and other neurologic problems. Since a screening test for detecting PKU in newborns was introduced in the 1960s, thousands of babies with PKU have been identified and put on phenylalanine-free diets to prevent brain damage. Most go off the diet without harm by the time they reach school age. (Phenylalanine is found in meat, fish, poultry, all milk products, eggs, nuts, and dried legumes.)

If women with PKU become pregnant, they face a new danger: their fetuses can suffer from the build-up of phenylalanine, which the mothers remain unable to metabolize. In one study, women with PKU had a much higher incidence of miscarriages and of babies with very small brains, mental retardation, and heart defects.

There are many unanswered questions about the risks of PKU in pregnancy. Some obstetricians believe that a phenylalanine-free diet can eliminate the risks to the fetus. The few studies that have been done have shown that a baby's growth and intelligence are more likely to be normal if the mother avoids phenylalanine from the beginning of pregnancy.

A simple blood test of phenylalanine levels can determine if you have PKU and if a child you conceive may be at risk. A genetic counselor can explain the odds of a baby inheriting this autosomal recessive disorder, and your obstetrician can describe the recommended diet.

Counseling

Genetic counselors cannot provide easy answers to all parents at risk. However, they can offer the facts and understanding that parents need to make informed, responsible decisions about having a child or continuing a pregnancy.

For couples who fear that their genetic makeup may jeopardize the well-being of their unborn children, counseling may be one of the most important experiences of their lives. They can find out exactly what has gone wrong in the past and why, what the odds are of the same error occurring again, if they are at risk for any future problems, and what prenatal tests, if any, are available. "I used to think that the worst thing that could happen would be finding out I'd conceived a child with a genetic defect," comments one woman who sought counseling after she became pregnant at age 39. "Now I realize that there's one thing worse: not finding out and living in fear until the baby's born."

5 . Is My Baby All Right?
Tests That Tell

"WILL MY BABY be all right?"

It is the question of every mother-to-be, asked in fear of knowing too much and in far greater fear of not knowing enough. Boy or girl, blond or brunette, blue eyes or brown—such distinctions seem trivial when the baby is still faceless, nameless, and sexless. "Just let it be normal," the parents pray, yearning for reassurance.

In the past, obstetricians had little to offer *but* words of reassurance. Very often there was no scientific way of answering questions about an unborn baby. Today, with new understanding of the world within the womb and an array of innovative tools and techniques, doctors can give a baby its first medical checkup long before its birth. And because of their improved ability in diagnosing potential problems, they can provide more effective care to babies in jeopardy before and during birth.

Each of the prenatal tests described in this chapter offers a different perspective of the developing fetus, but none provides enough information to answer all the questions physicians or parents might ask. That's why a combination of tests frequently is necessary, each carefully timed and coordinated so the various results come together like pieces in a puzzle. Yet, even with more data than might have been thought possible several years ago, the decision about what is best for your baby may be unclear. Ultimately your doctor's own clinical judgment plays the critical role in interpreting test results and deciding on appropriate treatment. And, since some of the diagnostic tests involve potential risks as well as benefits, your obstetrician also must weigh the possibility of complications against the urgency of the need to know more about what is happening within your womb. In this chapter we will describe current diagnostic techniques, the tests that check on a baby's well-being before birth, and the ways in which a baby's condition is monitored during labor and delivery.

· Diagnostic Procedures

Ultrasound (Sonography)

Ultrasound uses short pulses of high-frequency, low-intensity sound waves (above the normal range of hearing) to create images. It was first employed in industry to detect flaws in construction and during World War II to locate submarines below the ocean surface. As the sound waves echo off structures within your body, they are converted into electrical signals and transformed into images on a display screen. A physician with specialized training evaluates the sonographic images and photographs them for further analysis.

Why Ultrasound Is Performed Ultrasound can rule out or confirm potential problems, eliminating the need for additional testing procedures that may be hazardous to you or your baby. It can confirm a pregnancy within a few weeks of conception and is the definitive

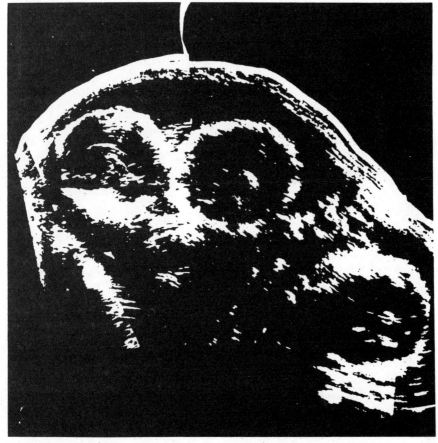

A sonogram of triplets

means of determining whether you are carrying more than one baby.

Obstetricians use ultrasound to diagnose a miscarriage or a misplaced (ectopic) pregnancy or to detect fetal malformations, including limb abnormalities, hydrocephalus (excessive fluid within the skull), some congenital heart and kidney defects, and excessive or insufficient amniotic fluid. It is the best method for examining the placenta's size, shape, and location; such information may be critical in pregnancies complicated by diabetes, Rh incompatibility, or growth problems. If bleeding from the vagina occurs in the last trimester, ultrasound may show whether the placenta is blocking the baby's way out of the uterus (a condition called placenta previa) or whether the placenta is separating from the uterine wall too soon (placental abruption).

Used early enough, particularly in high-risk pregnancies or if there is a problem in "dating" a pregnancy, ultrasound is a valuable tool for determining fetal age. From the eighth to the sixteenth week, ultrasound measurements of the distance from your baby's head to its rump or of the length of its femur (thigh bone) accurately indicate its gestational age. Later in pregnancy, measurement of the diameter of your baby's head (biparietal diameter) can indicate gestational age within one or two weeks. After twenty-nine weeks, there is such great biological variability in the way babies grow that sonographic measurements are not very helpful in dating the pregnancy.

Repeated, or serial, sonograms may be used to check on how your baby is growing. Measurements of the head and abdominal circumference made at intervals of two to four weeks can indicate whether a baby will be small or large for its gestational age. A special kind of ultrasound called real-time sonography can monitor your baby's heartbeat, breathing movements, and arm and leg motions. Ultrasound confirmations of these normal activities can be reassuring signs that your baby is healthy.

What to Expect Ultrasound usually is performed at your doctor's office or as an outpatient procedure at a hospital. You can go home immediately after the test. No injections or drugs are involved. The images of the uterus and baby are clearer if your bladder is full during the examination, so you will be asked to drink several glasses of water and not to urinate before the test. You will be given a hospital gown to wear.

During the test, you lie on your back on an examining table, uncovered from the top of your abdomen to your hips. Mineral oil or a gel rubbed on your skin improves the transmission of sound waves, which are produced by a small device called a transducer. The test is painless, although your full bladder may make you slightly uncomfortable as the transducer is pressed against your skin. The complete procedure usually takes less than half an hour.

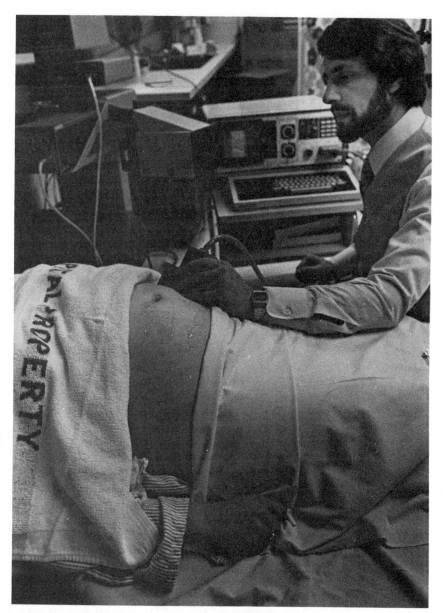

Radiologist Roy A. Filly, M.D., of the University of California, San Francisco, performs an ultrasonic examination *(David Powers)*

Concerns The benefits of the information provided by sonography are so great that obstetricians have described ultrasound as a "window into the womb" that has revolutionized their approach to prenatal care. While it is impossible to say that there are no risks at all, there have been no consistent reports of damage in the two decades in which ultrasound has been used extensively in pregnancy. Researchers are continuing to follow the development of babies who were examined before birth for any indication of possible harm. Until there is proof that it does not produce subtle or delayed harmful effects, ultrasound should be used only when medically indicated.

X-rays

Ultrasound has eliminated the need for almost all X-rays during pregnancy. On very rare occasions, amniography—X-ray visualization of the amniotic sac—may be used to detect suspected abnormalities of the soft tissues that do not show up clearly on sonograms. X-rays also may be necessary to diagnose some maternal problems, but they are avoided in the first trimester, when they are most harmful. The standard doses for such tests are not associated with an increased risk of congenital abnormalities. X-rays are occasionally used during labor for pelvimetry, a measurement of the pelvis to determine if the fetus will be able to pass through safely.

Amniocentesis

Amniocentesis is a method of removing a small amount of fluid from the amniotic sac for analysis. Developed in 1956, it initially helped obstetricians evaluate the condition of babies with Rh-incompatibility problems. Either the amniotic fluid itself or the cells that the fetus sheds into the fluid may be studied, depending on the reason for the test and the type of information needed.

Why Amniocentesis Is Performed As a genetic screening test (see Chapter 4), amniocentesis is recommended for women over age 35 because of the increased risk of Down's syndrome in their babies, for mothers who have borne a child with certain genetic and chromosomal abnormalities, for women who may be carriers of X-linked disorders, and for couples who both carry a recessive trait for a disease.

If a woman is sensitized to the Rh factor, amniocentesis can determine if the risks to her baby are increasing and if the fetus needs a transfusion of fresh red blood cells. The obstetrician analyzes the fluid for the amount of bilirubin, a yellowish pigment produced as a baby's red blood cells are destroyed by the mother's protective antibodies.

In the last weeks of pregnancy an obstetrician considering an early delivery may perform amniocentesis to determine if the unborn baby's lungs are sufficiently developed to function outside the womb. The levels of two critical substances—lecithin and sphingomyelin—in the amniotic fluid indicate whether the baby's lungs are mature (see page 51).

What to Expect Amniocentesis may be performed in a doctor's office or as an outpatient procedure in a hospital. It is not performed

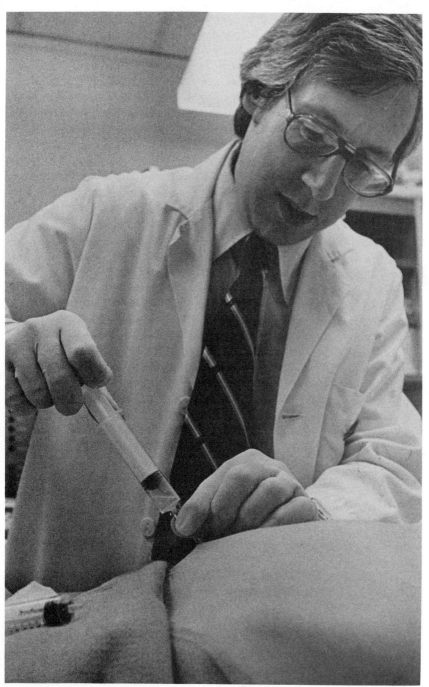

Mitchell S. Golbus, M.D., an obstetrician and geneticist at the University of California, San Francisco, performs amniocentesis to obtain fetal cells for chromosomal analysis *(Richard Brooks)*

before the twelfth week of pregnancy because the uterus cannot be felt through the abdominal wall before that time. Usually amniocentesis for genetic testing is scheduled for the sixteenth week, when the uterus can be located easily and a needle can be inserted into the amniotic sac without difficulty. Ultrasound before the procedure can pinpoint the exact location of the fetus and the placenta, which is particularly helpful in the first half of pregnancy. If amniocentesis is indicated in the last trimester, the doctor may be able to determine the baby's position by palpating your abdomen, making ultrasound unnecessary.

During the test, you lie on an examining table, your abdomen coated with an antiseptic solution to prevent infection. Local anesthesia is usually used; you will remain awake throughout the procedure. A thin needle, inserted through your skin into the amniotic sac, causes a sensation similar to that of an insect sting. About 5 to 15 milliliters of fluid—the equivalent of 3 tablespoons—is withdrawn, and a small Band-Aid is placed over the skin. The test, including preparation, usually takes less than ten minutes.

The sample is sent to a laboratory. For genetic studies, the fetal cells are grown in a nutrient broth. The fetal chromosomes are photographed and arranged into twenty-three pairs according to their size and structure. Sophisticated staining techniques, developed in the past decade, bring out patterns of light and dark bands, revealing subtle signs of genetic flaws. Careful examination indicates whether there are too many or too few chromosomes, whether some are out of place, if any are broken, and if certain segments are missing. Because the X and Y chromosomes are among those studied, it is possible to find out if the fetus is male or female. It takes several weeks for the fetal cells to multiply, so there is a delay of approximately four weeks before you receive the results of a chromosomal analysis.

In tests for metabolic disorders, such as neural tube defects, the fetal cells are grown in a tissue culture and analyzed for missing or abnormal enzymes. Blood abnormalities, such as some cases of sickle-cell disease and beta-thalassemia, also can be detected by analyzing the fetal cells. This process takes several weeks. In tests of Rh-related problems or lung maturity, the fluid itself is studied. This usually requires only a few hours, because the cells do not have to be specially prepared and grown.

Concerns The overall complication rate for amniocentesis is less than 1 percent. The risks are lower in the last trimester, when the amniotic sac is larger and easier to locate. There is a slight danger of miscarriage in the early part of pregnancy and of premature rupture of the membranes later in the pregnancy. Occasionally a physician draws a "bloody tap" because a maternal or, more rarely, fetal blood vessel is nicked. This generally does not cause serious problems.

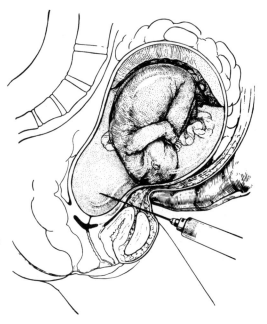

In the third trimester, amniocentesis may be performed to determine whether the baby is fully prepared for life outside the womb (Perinatal Care, *reprinted with permission*)

Fetoscopy

This still-experimental test is used in uncommon situations to answer questions that amniocentesis can not. Available at only a few medical centers, fetoscopy allows a physician to peer directly into the womb through a tube holding a light and special lenses (a fetoscope) and to obtain samples of an unborn baby's skin or blood.

Why Fetoscopy Is Performed Some serious congenital disorders, particularly blood abnormalities, cannot be diagnosed simply by growing fetal cells from the amniotic fluid. To detect these problems, physicians must obtain a sample of the baby's blood. If there is a *strong* possibility that a fetus has a grave blood or skin disorder that cannot be diagnosed by any other means, fetoscopy may be advised.

What to Expect Fetoscopy can be performed as an outpatient procedure. Ultrasound is used during the test to locate the fetus and placenta. To prevent infection, the doctor or nurse will coat your abdomen with an antiseptic and cover you with sterile surgical drapes. You will be given a local anesthetic. The physician makes a tiny incision, about 3 millimeters long, in the skin of your abdomen and inserts a sharp pointed instrument through the uterine wall into the amniotic sac; it contains the fetoscope. By means of light-transmitting fibers, he or she can see small areas of the fetus and can take photographs with special camera lenses. The doctor can also push a tiny forceps through the tube to take a minute sample of skin from the baby's scalp or use a miniscalpel to prick one of the fetal blood vessels in the placenta to obtain a few drops of blood for testing.

Concerns Fetoscopy is an experimental and delicate procedure with a complication rate of about 5 percent. The hazards to the fetus include miscarriage and bleeding; and the mother may be at risk if a blood vessel is punctured. Your physician will recommend this test only if the potential benefits clearly outweigh these risks.

• Tests of Your Baby's Well-Being in the Womb

Since an unborn baby has no way of letting you or your doctor know that something is wrong, your obstetrician relies on indirect methods of making sure that your baby is healthy.

Maternal Blood and Urine Tests

Throughout pregnancy, samples of your blood and urine provide information about your condition and your baby's well-being. Periodically your doctor will look for any signs of problems, such as infection, anemia, abnormal metabolism of food, and impaired clearance of fluids and wastes, and will measure certain proteins produced only during pregnancy, including estriol and placental lactogen.

Estriol Levels Estrogen increases markedly in pregnancy; the substance called estriol is the major component of the increased amount of this hormone. The fetus produces estriol precursors in its adrenal glands and converts them to estriol in its liver and in the placenta. Usually estriol levels in your blood and urine rise steadily throughout pregnancy. However, there is so much normal variation that several measurements over time are usually necessary to establish a trend.

Estriol levels that are normal for a given stage of your pregnancy are reassuring evidence that all is well within your womb. This can be very important information, particularly if you are diabetic or have hypertension. Estriol levels that are not increasing or that begin to fall may reflect danger to your baby. Yet it can be difficult to determine whether your baby is in jeopardy on the basis of estriol measurements alone. Sometimes, for example, estriol levels are low because of the administration of drugs, such as corticosteroids or antibiotics. Your doctor may suggest weekly testing of your estriol levels if you have hypertension, kidney disease, or pre-eclampsia (see Chapter 11 for an explanation of this blood pressure disorder). If you are diabetic, you may undergo daily tests of estriol late in your pregnancy. The reason is that in diabetics estriol levels may drop sharply over the course of just twenty-four to forty-eight hours, signaling an immediate threat to the baby's survival. If that happens, the obstetrician may perform other tests to confirm any danger or may choose to deliver the baby immediately.

Human Placental Lactogen (HPL) Levels HPL is a protein produced only in pregnancy. It increases in your bloodstream until about the thirty-seventh week and then levels off. Increases in HPL, like rises in estriol, provide reassurance of fetal well-being. Low HPL measurements are not a clear-cut sign of a problem but merely a hint of possible jeopardy. Other tests usually corroborate whether your baby is or is not doing well.

There is no danger to you or your baby from blood and urine tests of estriol and HPL, but you'll have to spend some extra time getting samples to your doctor or a laboratory. You may have to collect all of the urine you produce in a twenty-four period, store it in the refrigerator, and deliver it for laboratory testing. This may be inconvenient and time-consuming, but it provides valuable information about your baby.

Fetal Movements

One way of knowing if your baby is doing well inside the uterus in the final months of pregnancy is a test you can do by and for yourself: monitor its movements. Fetal activity is generally a reassuring sign of well-being. In the last trimester, you will clearly notice your baby's kicks and turns and dips—particularly when you are lying down. Once your baby's head settles into your pelvis in preparation for delivery, the movements will be less vigorous, but you will feel jabs from its arms and legs.

Every baby has its own daily pattern of activity, with periods of rest and of increased movement. A change from this pattern, particularly a marked decrease in activity, may be an indication of potential danger to your baby. A reduction in the number or intensity of fetal movements is a warning signal: about half of the babies who have a sudden, marked decrease or cessation of activity during a twelve-hour period die within twenty-four hours. Some of these losses might be prevented by immediate delivery.

In a high-risk pregnancy, your obstetrician may ask you to count your baby's movements regularly, sometimes as often as once or twice a day, beginning in your sixth month, Such self-monitoring is simple and reliable. You should set aside specific times for kick-counting so you'll be able to recognize any change from your baby's normal movement pattern. Lie down on your back or side. Pay careful attention to the sensations in your abdomen and count each movement. Three or more kicks in a two-hour period is considered normal. You can get up as soon as you detect three movements, but if your baby hasn't kicked three times in two hours, continue to lie still and count movements. If you detect fewer than ten kicks in a twelve-hour period, notify your obstetrician. If you feel no movements at all over twelve hours, your obstetrician may perform other tests to decide whether or not to go ahead with an immediate delivery. You also should report any sudden, substantive *increase* in activity.

Tests of Your Baby's Heart Rate

The two techniques most often used to monitor a baby's heart rate for subtle changes that may indicate problems are fetal heart-rate nonstress and stress tests. Both usually are performed in an office or labor room. They involve the use of an electronic monitor of your baby's heart and another device that records the frequency and duration of uterine contractions.

Nonstress Testing (NST) This test, which does not require any drugs or anesthesia, is painless and harmless for you and your baby. You lie in a hospital bed or on an examining table with an electronic monitoring device held around your abdomen by a belt (see page 53). For a period of about twenty minutes, your baby's heart rate and activity are recorded on a long, narrow strip of paper. A normal fetal heart rate is quite fast—about 120 to 160 beats per minute—and there is definite variability from one heartbeat to the next. If your baby moves or if your uterus contracts, the heart rate typically accelerates.

On the basis of its heart-rate pattern, your baby will be classified as "nonreactive" or "reactive." A reactive baby's heart speeds up in response to at least two movements or contractions during the twenty-minute period; this is a good sign that all is well. A nonreactive baby shows no variability between heartbeats and no speeding up of the heart with movement.

A nonreactive nonstress test is not a clear indication of risk, as only about 20 percent of nonreactive babies actually are in jeopardy. To get a more precise indication of the risk to your baby if the nonstress test is nonreactive, your doctor may perform a stress, or oxytocin challenge, test.

Stress Testing The procedure for a stress test is similar to what happens during nonstress evaluation. You lie in bed or on a table, connected to a monitor of your baby's heart and activity. The difference is that oxytocin, a hormone that stimulates uterine contractions (which "stress" or challenge your baby), is fed into your bloodstream through an intravenous (IV) tube. The dose increases gradually until contractions occur every three to four minutes for a period of fifteen to thirty minutes. Most women describe this test as mildly uncomfortable but not painful. The contractions are a challenge to the baby, similar to the challenge of normal labor. Since only a few contractions are induced, they do not have an adverse effect on a baby.

Stress testing can yield positive, negative, or inconclusive results. A positive result indicates potential danger, because the baby's heart slows down rather than speeds up in response to a contraction and does not return to normal until after a contraction is over (this is called a deceleration; see page 55). Your baby may react this way because of inadequate "reserve," or staying power, and therefore may be at higher risk during the rigorous process of labor. A negative stress test is a good sign that your baby is strong. In response to contractions, its heart rate speeds up, and there is good beat-to-beat variability. Sometimes the results are inconclusive, particularly if the baby does not show any consistent pattern of reacting to contractions.

Stress testing is considered more precise than nonstress tests, but there still is a high percentage of "false abnormals," and about 25 percent of babies with positive stress tests actually are healthy. Your doctor may repeat the procedure or use other tests, such as estriol levels and kick-counting, to double-check the results.

Lung Maturity Tests

If a combination of tests of fetal well-being indicates that your baby is in jeopardy in the womb, the best next step may be an early delivery. However, babies who are born before the natural term of pregnancy are more likely to develop respiratory distress syndrome (RDS), an often-fatal breathing difficulty associated with fragile, immature lungs. In the effort to balance the hazards of allowing the pregnancy to continue against the possible risk of RDS, your obstetrician will find out whether your baby's lungs have developed a crucial substance called surfactant, which is essential for breathing. This chemical lining of the tiny air sacs in the lungs usually is produced between the thirty-fourth and thirty-seventh weeks of pregnancy. Several tests can check surfactant production and lung maturity.

Lecithin/Sphingomyelin (L/S) Ratio Lecithin and sphingomyelin are two lipids (fats). Lecithin, a component of surfactant, is produced by the lungs; sphingomyelin is produced by the skin. During the first eight months of pregnancy, there are equal amounts of lecithin and sphingomyelin in the amniotic fluid. However, as the lungs complete their development they produce a sudden surge of lecithin, and the ratio of lecithin to sphingomyelin changes from one to one to two to one.

Your doctor can check your baby's L/S ratio by performing amniocentesis, so the L/S ratio in a sample of amniotic fluid can be computed. If it is less than two to one, the doctor may choose to delay delivery and initiate treatment with steroids, drugs that speed up lung maturation.

Shake Test A much quicker way of testing lung maturity is to place the sample of amniotic fluid in a test tube with an equal amount of alcohol and shake the mixture. If stable bubbles or a ring of foam appears, the risk of respiratory problems after birth is less than 0.5 percent. If bubbles do not form, the lungs may not have manufactured surfactant and may not be ready for life outside the womb. The fluid may be analyzed and the L/S ratio computed if the shake test is negative. There are also more elaborate assays that yield further information about the maturity of the baby's lungs.

· Tests During Labor and Delivery

Being born is a stressful and complex process. Every time the uterus contracts, the blood vessels that supply the baby with oxygen are constricted. In effect, the baby is forced to hold its breath. Healthy babies are able to do this without any problem, just as healthy adults can, but other babies are more vulnerable during labor. Like adults with chronic lung problems, they cannot hold their breath for an extended period. If deprived of oxygen for too long, they may suffer permanent neurological impairment or die. To avoid these devastating dangers, obstetricians monitor babies carefully throughout labor and delivery.

Meconium in the Amniotic Fluid

Meconium is a waste product of the unborn baby that is released into the amniotic fluid in about 10 percent of deliveries. The presence of meconium indicates fetal distress, possibly as a result of oxygen deprivation, and increased danger.

Meconium may be detected during amniocentesis performed to test for lung maturity, or when the membranes of the amniotic sac break. If only a small amount of meconium has been released, the fluid may simply have a greenish tinge. A more ominous sign is thick, heavy meconium. Babies with meconium in their amniotic fluid are closely watched with electronic monitors. A specialist in newborn care may be present at the delivery to begin immediate treatment.

Meconium is a direct threat to the baby, who may inhale (aspirate) it either in the womb or shortly after delivery. The nose, throat, and breathing passages must be suctioned immediately to prevent respiratory problems, including pneumonia.

Electronic Fetal Monitoring

An unusual fetal heart rate can signal distress and danger. In the past, physicians and nurses monitored a baby's heart by listening through a stethoscope pressed against the mother's abdomen at regular intervals during labor. In 1969 the electronic fetal monitor was introduced to provide continuous surveillance of the baby's heart rate and of uterine contractions. Its use has had an enormous impact on obstetricians' approach to complications during delivery. The widespread reliance on fetal monitors also has set off a nationwide controversy among obstetricians and their patients. Electronic monitoring has been criticized as unnecessary in low-risk births, but there is little disagreement about the value of close surveillance in complicated or high-risk deliveries.

At some hospitals, all women in labor are monitored at least initially or at regular intervals during labor. If there are any signs that the baby may be in distress, electronic fetal monitoring continues throughout labor and delivery.

What to Expect There are two types of electronic fetal monitoring: external and internal. In external monitoring, the instruments are all outside the body. Two belts are placed around the abdomen. One holds a small instrument, called a tocotransducer, that records the tightness and stretch of your abdomen during contractions and tells how long and how far apart the contractions are. The other belt holds an ultrasound transducer that records your baby's heart rate. These belts are generally comfortable and don't interfere with labor.

Once your amniotic membranes rupture and your cervix opens to at least 1 centimeter, one or both of the external monitors may be replaced by more sensitive and accurate internal devices placed directly in your womb. An electrode attached to the baby's scalp can produce a fetal electrocardiogram, a record of its heartbeat. A fluid-filled plastic tube also may be placed in your uterus; it records the pressure within your uterus during contractions.

A trained nurse will be in your room, caring for you as well as

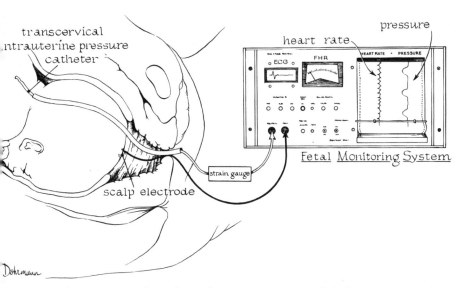

In internal monitoring, electrodes and gauges monitor the baby's heart rate and the pressure of contractions during labor

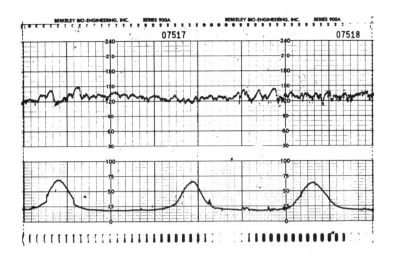

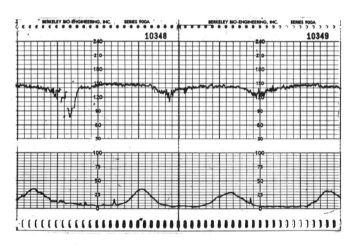

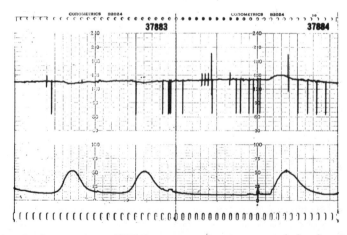

Electronic fetal monitoring (EFM) patterns, showing normal deceleration; late deceleration; lack of beat-to-beat variability

watching the monitor. Your doctor also will check the tracings while evaluating your progress in labor.

What Monitoring Indicates The electronic fetal monitor records both uterine contractions and the baby's electrocardiogram on a continuous paper printout much like an adult electrocardiogram (EKG). In evaluating these tracings, your obstetrician looks for any abnormal heart-rate patterns.

A normal pattern has a jagged, sawtooth appearance because of the typical variation between heartbeats. A flattened tracing may be the result of pain-relief medications, and the baby may be fine. But it also may indicate oxygen deprivation. During a contraction, the heart rate of a healthy baby accelerates or stays the same. If a baby is in distress, its heart rate decelerates, or slows down briefly. There are three types of periodic decelerations that may occur:

• Early decelerations begin at the same time as a contraction and stop when the contraction stops. They are not considered ominous.

• Late decelerations begin after the onset of a contraction. About 50 percent of the time they are related to oxygen deprivation. Sometimes they can be stopped if the mother changes position or inhales oxygen.

• Variable decelerations are just that—variable in shape, time of onset, and duration. They usually represent compression of the umbilical cord; and the longer, more persistent, and more intense they are, the greater the likelihood of fetal distress.

Concerns A major problem with electronic fetal monitoring is interpretation of the tracings of the baby's heart rate. The great majority of babies do not show abnormal heart patterns during labor, yet not all babies with unusual heart rates are actually in distress. When electronic monitors were introduced, obstetricians were criticized for reacting too quickly and aggressively to any variation in a baby's heart rate and treating the delivery as an emergency situation. Experience with the equipment has overcome this problem. When an obstetrician is unsure if a heart tracing is ominous, he or she can use another test—fetal scalp sampling—to get a better idea of the baby's condition.

Fetal Scalp Sampling

If your baby's heart rate is abnormal, your obstetrician may need to analyze a blood sample for more information. After your membranes have ruptured, he or she will insert an amnioscope (a cone-shaped device with an attached light source) into your vagina to view the baby's presenting part, usually its head. After cleansing the scalp, the doctor pricks one of the tiny blood vessels. The blood is analyzed quickly to measure its pH, an indication of the acidity of the blood, and PCO_2, a measurement of carbon dioxide in the blood. A baby with a high PCO_2

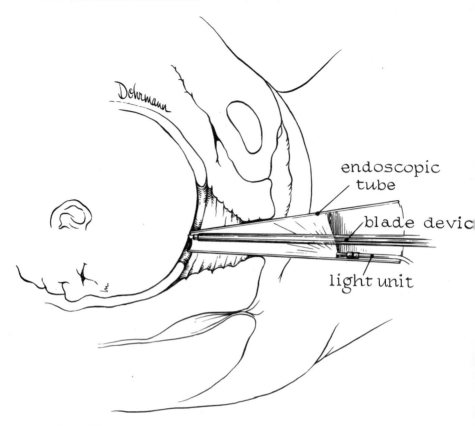

Dohrmann

endoscopic
tube

blade devic

light unit

Scalp sampling is used to get more precise information about a baby's condition prior to birth

is usually suffering from oxygen deprivation and may be delivered immediately.

Scalp sampling is usually performed only if the fetal heart rate shows possible signs of distress. There is a complication rate of less than 1 percent, including fetal bleeding or an abcess on the scalp.

6 . *Protecting Your Baby: Drugs and Chemicals*

BABY JONES flails her arms in awkward, jerking motions. Her mouth opens in a cry, but her voice is so weak that the sound cannot be heard a few yards away. Her skin seems too big for her skeleton; she looks wrinkled and oddly old. The first days of Baby Jones's life have been exceptionally hard. Much smaller than most newborns, she has had problems feeding, breathing, and maintaining her body temperature. The neonatologists think she'll pull through, but they fear that the day she leaves the intensive-care nursery will not be the end of a difficult beginning, but the beginning of a difficult life. Baby Jones will never be as bright or as tall or as capable as she might have been. Her life will be shadowed forever by events that occurred before her birth—events that could have been prevented if her mother had stopped drinking heavily while pregnant.

One of every 750 babies in the United States is born, as Baby Jones was, with fetal alcohol syndrome, a cluster of physical and mental defects associated with chronic alcoholism. And alcohol, the most socially acceptable drug in our society, is far from the only one that is used—and abused—by pregnant women. According to some estimates, drugs and chemicals may be responsible, at least in part, for 25 percent of congenital malformations and 15 percent of perinatal deaths. But so little is known about the effects that most substances have on an unborn baby that scientists cannot be sure whether these estimates are far too high or far too low.

Statistics seem somewhat beside the point when thinking about infants like Baby Jones, or the "thalidomide babies" of the 1960s who were born with limb defects, or the "DES daughters" whose mothers were given diethylstilbestrol during their pregnancies. It is too late to help any of these individuals, for the damage that occurred before their births is irreversible. However, their plight put physicians and pregnant women on the alert. Learning from these problems of the past, researchers have investigated the ways in which drugs of every type—prescription and nonprescription, legal and illegal—may interfere with fetal development. And a new philosophy toward drugs in pregnancy has evolved, one based on the premise that no drug should be prescribed or used unless its benefits outweigh its potential risks.

· Understanding the Risks

Any substance that causes deformities in an unborn baby is called a teratogen, from the Latin word *terato* for monster. Some teratogens have such devastating effects that they destroy the embryo or trigger a miscarriage. Others have an impact so subtle that it may not be noticed for several years or even decades. Teratogens have different effects at different stages of pregnancy. In the initial seventeen days from the time of fertilization, the cells are reproducing rapidly. Exposure to a toxic (harmful) substance during this period interferes with all the cells, resulting in the death of the developing organism even before the mother may suspect that she is pregnant. From the seventeenth to the fifty-fifth day after fertilization, the major organs needed to sustain life begin to develop. A teratogen can damage cells as they are specializing and, therefore, can affect an entire organ or set of organs. This is the period in which most major birth defects begin. After the fifty-fifth day of gestation, the basic development of fetal organs is complete. Exposure to a toxin in the second or third trimester generally does not cause major defects but can interfere with normal growth and development and may affect a baby's well-being during and immediately after birth.

Certain drugs pose less of a threat later in pregnancy; others become more hazardous. Taken in high doses in the final weeks before delivery, aspirin—which is not considered harmful early in pregnancy—may impair fetal circulation, prolong the duration of pregnancy, and increase bleeding by both mother and baby during delivery. The risks of a drug like alcohol are different early and late in pregnancy. Many of the destructive effects of fetal alcohol syndrome begin in the first trimester. Heavy drinking in the last trimester alone depresses a baby's normal responsiveness during and after birth.

According to the National Institutes of Health Collaborative Perinatal Study, 65 percent of pregnant women take drugs—prescription or nonprescription—on their own; the average number of drugs taken per woman is 1.5. But throughout pregnancy self-medication can do more harm than good.

From the time you discover you're pregnant until your baby is born, you shouldn't take *any* drug without your doctor's permission. Many people don't think they're using drugs when they drink coffee or smoke cigarettes, but caffeine and nicotine can affect your baby's health and growth. Nonprescription drugs, such as aspirin or laxatives, can have as much impact as prescription medications. That's why you should always check with your obstetrician first.

In this chapter we will review what is known about the possible dangers of alcohol, nicotine, caffeine, food additives, illicit drugs, and nonprescription remedies. And we will also describe the relative benefits and risks of the drugs most frequently prescribed during pregnancy.

• Alcohol

The Old Testament admonished women to "drink no wine or strong drink" before bearing a child. In early Carthage, newlyweds were forbidden to drink on their wedding night for fear that they might conceive a defective child. In what may be the earliest medical report on alcoholism in pregnancy, British physicians in the late 1800s noted a higher incidence of stillborn or very sick babies among women jailed for drunkenness in Liverpool. Yet, despite such long-standing concern, only in the last decade have large-scale studies documented that alcohol does indeed cause disorders such as mental retardation, growth impairment, brain and nervous system abnormalities, and death in the womb.

Alcohol is a particularly dangerous teratogen because it passes freely across the placenta, reaching concentrations in the fetal blood as high as in the mother's. Its effects increase along with the amount that a mother-to-be drinks. Babies of women who are chronic alcoholics face a 30 to 50 percent risk of being born with fetal alcohol syndrome. Regardless of their race or ethnic background, infants with this set of congenital abnormalities look remarkably alike. They have short eye slits, a low nose bridge, ridges running between the nose and mouth, a narrow upper lip, a small chin, and a flat look to their faces. Sometimes they have drooping eyelids or crossed eyes, and they're likely to have minor abnormalities of their joints and genitals and unusual crease patterns in the palms of their hands. About 30 percent have heart defects. They are shorter and smaller than most newborns, with significantly smaller brains. Irritable as infants, they grow up to be hyperactive children with retarded mental and motor development. Their average IQ is about 68 (mildly retarded). Even when children with fetal alcohol syndrome have been placed in nurturing environments and given excellent opportunities for education, most have shown no significant improvement.

The risk of fetal alcohol syndrome is greatest if a mother drinks 3 or more ounces of pure alcohol (the equivalent of six or more cocktails) a day. (One ounce of standard-proof whiskey is equal to ½ ounce of pure alcohol.) Milder but similar problems occur in about 10 percent of the babies born to women who consume 1 to 2 ounces (two to four cocktails) a day.

Does that mean a single drink a day is safe? Not necessarily. The dangers of moderate drinking—a cocktail or glass of wine every day, for example—are not firmly established. Some researchers have linked an ounce of alcohol a day to low birth weights and 2 ounces a week to an increased miscarriage rate. The National Institute on Alcohol Abuse and Alcoholism and the U.S. Surgeon General advise pregnant women, and those trying to become pregnant, to avoid all alcohol. This recommendation is based not on research data implicating limited drinking, but on the premise that the only way to avoid all the potential dangers of alcohol is to avoid all alcohol. An *occasional* glass of wine is not likely to cause any harm to your baby.

• Nicotine

Smoking during pregnancy jeopardizes the well-being of two individuals—you and the baby developing in your smoke-filled womb. The major danger for the baby is growth retardation. Regardless of their prepregnancy weight or how many pounds they put on during pregnancy, smokers tend to have babies that weigh 150 to 170 grams (5¼ to 6 ounces) less than normal. Smoking also has been associated with placental abruptions (premature separation of the placenta from the wall of the uterus).

The risks to your baby increase with the number of cigarettes you smoke. You can overcome potential dangers by cutting back or, preferably, quitting. Because your baby grows most rapidly in the final trimester, it will have a good chance of attaining a normal birth weight if you stop smoking as late as the final three months. Even quitting a short time before delivery can help. A study in Wales demonstrated that women who stopped smoking in the forty-eight hours prior to delivery had more oxygen reserve than mothers who continued to smoke until labor began.

• Caffeine

Caffeine belongs to a chemical family called the xanthines, which include the compounds found in chocolate, cocoa, cola, and tea. When you drink coffee while pregnant, you expose your baby to the same concentration of caffeine as is in your own blood. The caffeine equivalent of five or six cups of coffee a day increases the risk of birth defects in laboratory animals. It is not clear whether the same effect might occur in human beings, but caffeine may increase the risk of stillbirths, miscarriages, and preterm labor. One study of pregnant women who were heavy coffee drinkers found a higher incidence of these complications; another study found no clear link. The Food and Drug Administration (FDA) has recommended that women who are or are trying to become pregnant avoid or limit their consumptions of foods and drugs containing caffeine although researchers have not been able to prove a conclusive risk of any damage to the unborn baby.

You may want to refer to the following checklist of caffeine-containing substances in evaluating your caffeine intake.

Product	Mg Caffeine
Cup of coffee	75–155 mg
Cup of tea	90–150 mg
12 oz. cola drink	30–65 mg
Cup of cocoa	2–40 mg
1 oz. solid milk chocolate	6 mg
Over-the-counter stimulant	100–200 mg

(SOURCE: *FDA Drug Bulletin*, Vol. 10, No. 3, November 1980)

· Food Additives

Food additives are chemicals added to foods to fortify them with more nutrients, enrich them with nutrients lost in processing, prevent the growth of bacteria and fungi, or color or flavor the foods. Some additives have nutritive value and are considered beneficial; many are safe for you and your baby. You should avoid or limit the use of others because of possible harm to your baby. The list of food additives in Appendix may help you eat a bit more wisely during pregnancy. Keep in mind that there is no evidence of a cause-and-effect relationship between additives and harm to your baby.

· Illicit Drugs

Very little is known about the effects of nonnarcotic street drugs, such as marijuana and cocaine, during pregnancy. While no studies have been done to prove that they are harmful, neither is there any evidence that they are safe. To avoid potential risks, you should avoid them entirely. Research into the effects of lysergic acid (LSD) suggests some increased risk of limb and nervous system defects in the children of women who take LSD while pregnant. There is no evidence of chromosomal damage or breakage in women who used LSD prior to conception.

Narcotics are known threats to an unborn child. A baby of a woman addicted to heroin is at much greater risk of growth impairment and preterm births. In addition, about 65 to 70 percent of the babies of narcotic users become addicted in the womb. After delivery they undergo a painful and precarious withdrawal process, which proves fatal for 3 to 5 percent of these infants.

• Nonprescription Drugs

Many people don't consider over-the-counter medications "real" drugs because they can be obtained without a prescription. However, these compounds do contain powerful chemicals that could affect your growing baby. You should never take *any* medication without consulting your doctor. This includes such widely used drugs as:

• *Aspirin.* Probably taken more often than any other medicine in the world, aspirin can cause a variety of complications for you and your baby if taken in large doses in your last trimester. The evidence on its effects, while not conclusive, suggests that aspirin may prolong gestation, increase the duration of labor, increase fetal and maternal bleeding at delivery, and interfere with fetal circulation.

• *Antinausea medications.* Many of these drugs have antihistamines as their primary ingredient. You should check with your doctor before taking them. The nausea and vomiting common in early pregnancy usually can be relieved by eating smaller meals and avoiding spicy foods. While there are no known dangers with such stomach-soothing antacid drugs as Mylanta and Maalox, you should check with your doctor before using them.

• *Laxatives.* Rather than relying on medication for constipation, drink more fluids and eat high-fiber foods, such as bran and fresh fruits. Do not use mineral oil because it decreases vitamin absorption by you and your baby.

• *Cough and cold preparations.* Little research has been done on the safety of cold remedies, which often contain a combination of ingredients, during pregnancy. Use them only as directed by your doctor.

• *Antihistamines.* These drugs, which counteract a powerful body chemical called histamine that produces many of the uncomfortable symptoms of colds or allergies, are common ingredients in cough and cold remedies, sleeping pills, and antinausea preparations.

Because some over-the-counter medications contain significant amounts of antihistamines, your doctor may advise you to avoid specific medications or may limit the dose.

• *Sleeping aids.* You may have difficulty sleeping, particularly late in your pregnancy, because of your baby's movements and your need to urinate frequently. Over-the-counter sleep aids, many of which have not been tested in pregnancy, contain significant amounts of antihistamines and have limited effectiveness at any time; they cannot solve these problems and should be avoided.

• *Vitamins and minerals.* *Williams Obstetrics*, the "bible" of obstetricians, describes the use of prenatal vitamin supplements as "a deeply engrained habit of many obstetricians, even though scientific evidence to show that the usual vitamin supplements are of benefit to either the mother or her fetus is quite meager. The Committee on Maternal Nutrition of the National Research Council pointed out that, in the majority of cases, routine pharmaceutical supplementation of vitamin and mineral preparations to pregnant women is of doubtful value, except for iron and possibly folic acid." The committee emphasized that no vitamin should be regarded as a substitute for food and a nutritious, well-balanced diet.

Very high doses of certain vitamins actually can be too much of a good thing. Excessive amounts of vitamin A have been associated with kidney abnormalities. Very high doses of vitamin D in the first trimester have been linked with mental retardation. Daily doses of more than a gram of vitamin C also can lead to problems for the baby after birth.

The two supplements that are recommended are folic acid and iron; both help to prevent anemia. Combination tablets, consisting of 30 to 60 milligrams of iron plus .3 to 1 milligram of folic acid, are most commonly prescribed.

Your doctor should advise you on what dosage form and strength are best for you.

• Prescription Drugs

The only medicines you should take while pregnant are those that are absolutely essential for you or your baby's well-being. Your obstetrician will balance the potential benefits of a drug against the possible risks to your baby. Sometimes that decision is clear-cut, because not treating an illness is much more hazardous than the potential complications related to treatment. However, choosing the appropriate medication and an effective but safe dose can be a therapeutic challenge.

Relatively few prescription drugs have been *proven* to be teratogens. However, most have not been tested to confirm or rule out the possibility of harm. Since 1980 the Food and Drug Administration has required that all prescription medications be labeled according to their potential effects during pregnancy. The FDA classification system is explained in the chart on page 64.

The specific drugs used to treat specific problems are discussed in the chapters on medical problems in Part 2. The following list includes some of the most commonly prescribed categories of drugs and indicates which medications are considered to be harmful or potentially harmful, which have been proven safe, and which have not been proven to be either dangerous or safe.

FDA CATEGORIES FOR PRESCRIPTION DRUG USE IN PREGNANCY

The Food and Drug Administration requires drug manufacturers to label all prescription medications to indicate whether they are safe to an unborn baby. The following FDA categories include designations of proved safety (Category A) and definite risk (Category X). The labels for categories B and C are not as clear, either because of a lack of research on the drug's effects in humans or contradictory results in tests with animals and with human beings. The drugs placed in Category D entail a definite risk, but their potential benefits are considered greater than their potential for harm.

Category A

The possibility of fetal harm as a result of use of these drugs seems remote. Controlled studies in women have shown no risk at any point in pregnancy.

Category B

These drugs have not been proved dangerous, but the research is not considered conclusive. There may not be any controlled studies of pregnant women, but laboratory experiments with animals have not demonstrated any risk. Conversely, controlled studies of pregnant women have revealed no risk, although animal research has indicated some adverse effect.

Category C

These drugs should be used only if the potential benefits clearly outweigh the proved possibility of risk. The assessment of potential risk may be based on animal studies showing adverse effects or may reflect a lack of research data from animal and human studies.

Category D

These drugs definitely pose a risk to an unborn baby, and there will be a warning on the drug label. However, these medications may be needed during pregnancy for the sake of the mother's well-being. For example, the drug may be needed in a life-threatening situation or for a disease for which there are no safer effective drugs.

Category X

The risk to a developing baby is too great to warrant the use of these drugs in pregnancy. A label on the drug package will state that the drug is "contraindicated" (should not be used) in women who are pregnant or who are trying to become pregnant. The assessment of risk is based on studies in animals or human beings that demonstrated fetal abnormalities or on direct evidence from human experience.

Drugs to Fight Infections (Antibiotics and Antimicrobials)

Penicillin and its derivatives, which have no known adverse effects on a fetus, are used most often for bacterial infections in pregnancy. The sulfonamides also are considered safe in humans, though they are usually not given immediately prior to delivery because they may cause jaundice (a buildup of bilirubin) in some newborns. Several antibiotics are not prescribed during pregnancy because of their teratogenic effects: Streptomycin can cause hearing loss and abnormally short or small limbs. Tetracycline can inhibit bone growth and discolor the tiny buds that eventually become teeth. Gentamicin and kanamycin may cause hearing impairment or loss.

Drugs to Prevent Blood Clots (Anticoagulants)

Heparin is the drug most commonly used for blood clotting problems in pregnant women. It is considered safe for the fetus, but must be taken by injection. Other anticlotting medications—warfarin and bishydroxycoumarin—are considered too hazardous to the fetus. About 25 to 50 percent of the babies whose mothers receive these latter drugs are born with bone defects, short hands, eye problems, and mental retardation. Chapter 12 discusses the risks of blood clots and the benefits of treatment in greater detail.

Drugs for Seizure Disorders (Anticonvulsants)

A syndrome of birth defects, including altered facial features, growth deficiency, mental retardation, cleft lip and palate, and cardiac anomalies, is associated with some anticonvulsants. Physicians therefore avoid the use of two drugs—trimethadione and paramethadione—during pregnancy. Barbiturates, which seem less likely to cause birth defects, are generally preferred in pregnancy, but sometimes only phenytoin (Dilantin) is effective in controlling seizures. If it is used, there is a 90 to 95 percent likelihood that the baby will be completely normal. If you are taking an anticonvulsant for a seizure disorder, your doctor will monitor the levels of the drug in your blood, keeping doses as low as possible to minimize risks to your baby. Treatment for a seizure disorder is always tailored to individual needs. Chapter 15 includes more information on the risks of seizures and the options for controlling them.

Magnesium sulfate is used to prevent or control seizures in women who develop severe high blood pressure complications, such as preeclampsia and eclampsia (see Chapter 11). It is not considered dangerous to the fetus.

Drugs for Respiratory Problems

Specific antihistamines prescribed to relieve allergies have no confirmed adverse effects on the fetus. Terbutaline and theophylline, both used to treat asthma, are also considered safe. Isoniazid, a treatment for tuberculosis, has been associated with increased anomalies in animal studies; rifampin is preferred because human studies have shown no teratogenic effects, although some abnormalities did occur in research animals.

Drugs to Control Diabetes

Insulin is considered safe throughout pregnancy, although doses may have to be readjusted frequently (see Chapter 13). Tolbutamide and chlorpropamide, oral medications for diabetics, cause an overall increase in fetal anomalies and should be avoided.

Drugs for Lowering Blood Pressure

Diuretics (drugs that increase urine production) are the basic treatment of chronic hypertension. If initiated before midpregnancy, they can be used safely until delivery. If given later in pregnancy, diuretics can decrease the mother's blood volume for one to three weeks before it returns to normal. This could endanger the baby, so obstetricians generally do not prescribe diuretics for the first time once the twentieth week of gestation has passed.

Hydralazine is an antihypertensive medication that has been linked with anomalies in animals but is considered safe in humans. Reserpine can cause breathing difficulties in newborns and is avoided late in pregnancy. Methyldopa has no known complications for the fetus. Propranolol may cause temperature regulation problems in newborns and may decrease the output of blood from the fetal heart. All of these medications should be used only under close medical observation and direction.

Drugs for Skin Disorders

Podophyllin, which is used topically to treat warts, may harm a developing fetus. You should avoid its use during pregnancy. Ointments for relief of itching or rashes should be used only as your doctor directs.

Drugs for Digestive Problems

The drug used most often over the past twenty years for nausea and vomiting in early pregnancy is doxylamine (Bendectin). Legal claims have asserted that Bendectin is teratogenic. The FDA, after reviewing the risks and benefits of the drug, concluded that available studies do not demonstrate an increased risk of birth defects, but that there is some "residual uncertainty" about Bendectin's absolute safety. While research continues, the FDA has recommended that Bendectin be prescribed only for severe cases of nausea and vomiting.

Drugs for Psychiatric Problems

Your obstetrician, consulting with your psychiatrist, will weigh the need to continue psychoactive medications during pregnancy. Although animal studies have linked antidepressant drugs with limb and central nervous system anomalies, the various medications for depression—haloperidol, the tricyclics, monoamine oxidase (MAO) inhibitors, and imipramine—generally provide benefits that outweigh possible risks. Lithium, a drug used for certain types of depression, is not frequently used in pregnancy because it causes birth defects in animals; in the last trimester, it may slow the baby's heart rate, lower its temperature and depress its central nervous system. Chronic use of two of the most widely prescribed antianxiety drugs in the Western world—the benzodiazepines better known by their trade names, Valium and Librium—has been associated with a possible but slight increase in cleft palate and heart defects in animals. Meprobamate (Miltown) carries many of the same associations. If these sedatives are used in the last trimester, the baby may suffer withdrawal symptoms after birth.

Drugs for Thyroid Problems

Iodides, the standard treatment for hyperthyroidism (excess production of thyroid hormone), are not used in pregnancy because of the danger of goiters, hypothyroidism (inadequate thyroid levels), and mental retardation in the newborn. The risk-benefit ratio for another agent, propylthiouracil, warrants its use, although there is a potential risk of goiter if high doses are given late in pregnancy.

Thyroid extracts for a hypothyroid mother do not cross the placenta. They maintain normal thyroid levels in the mother, and so are beneficial to her and her baby.

Hormones

Synthetic forms of estrogen and progesterone, previously used to prevent miscarriage, have been linked with anomalies. Diethylstilbestrol (DES), used in the 1940s and 1950s, caused genital anomalies in the sons and daughters of the women who were given it. Continued use of oral contraceptives early in pregnancy slightly increases the risk of heart and limb malformations. The corticosteroids, including topical preparations, have caused cleft palate in animal studies, in the first trimester; this has never been a problem in humans. They are associated with a minimal reduction in the weight of the baby if taken later in pregnancy.

• Radiation

The unborn children of women exposed to the intense radiation of the atomic bomb explosions in Japan in World War II suffered multiple effects, including an increased incidence of leukemia, thyroid tumors, and a variety of adult cancers. High levels of radiation of the type used for cancer therapy have been associated with birth defects, particularly incomplete brain development and mental deficiency.

Diagnostic X-rays are not considered a significant threat to the unborn. Doses of less than one roentgen are similar to normal background radiation. Absorption of one to ten roentgens from the second to the sixteenth week of pregnancy may be associated with malformations, but the danger is not considered so grave that abortion would be advised. Doses of more than ten roentgens in the first trimester would involve a much greater probability of damage, and the mother is usually advised to consider abortion. An individual may face increased risk of leukemia in later life if exposed to X-rays before birth. The risk at most is twice that of normal background radiation, which varies from place to place, but still is quite low. If the risk in an area is one in four thousand, the increased risk with X-rays would be one in two thousand.

· Environmental and Occupational Chemicals

Very little is known about an unborn baby's vulnerability to pollutants, toxic wastes, heavy metals, pesticides, gases, or synthetic compounds. There have been isolated reports—but no well-documented studies— that lead and cadmium are hazardous to a fetus, that pesticides like DDT can be found in the breast milk of women who live near sprayed areas, and that on-the-job exposure to chemicals such as kepone and DBCP may increase the risks of birth defects.

The most extensive studies of occupational risks have focused on physicians and nurses exposed daily to anesthetic gases. The results showed a higher incidence of miscarriages and congenital malformations in the babies of operating-room nurses, female anesthesiologists, and the wives of male anesthesiologists. Other research has found similar problems in female dentists and the wives of dentists who regularly used anesthetic gas in their practices.

Because so little research has been done on environmental and occupational risks to the fetus there are no well-established guidelines for employers or employees to follow in safeguarding the unborn. If you work in a setting that may be dangerous, consult your doctor or call the local office of the Occupational Safety and Health Agency (OSHA) to get information on specific chemicals or gases.

· Prevention and Protection

Teratogens pose many difficult issues—not only for you as a prospective parent, but for everyone concerned about the well-being of the next generation.

The extent of scientific understanding of these dangers is quite limited, in part because it often is almost impossible to pinpoint exactly how a baby is affected before birth. During the period of greatest susceptibility (the first trimester), a variety of causes—genetic, chemical, or environmental—can produce the same malformation. Very often a single teratogen will lead to multiple anomalies, rather than just one. There also seems to be a genetically determined vulnerability to harm.

If two fetuses are exposed to the same doses of a chemical at the same time, one may be severely deformed while the other may develop only a mild disorder or none at all. Most birth defects seem to involve an interaction of genetic and environmental factors. This makes it all the more difficult to isolate one cause of a problem or cluster of problems.

In a society that uses as many drugs and produces as many chemicals as ours, the prospect of safeguarding your unborn baby may seem intimidating. Again, it is important to keep these risks in perspective. You can do a great deal to prevent certain problems—by not smoking, not drinking alcohol, and not eating or drinking potentially harmful substances. If you develop a medical problem, it is in your baby's best interest as well as yours to seek appropriate treatment. If you're concerned about potential risks of medications, talk to your doctor and pharmacist about what is known about the effects of the drugs in question.

In a sense, you can protect your unborn baby exactly as you would any other child. You wouldn't give an infant a drink, a cigarette, a cup of coffee, or the pills you're taking for a medical complaint. You'd also be careful of the environment in which your child plays and of the foods he or she eats. Before birth, as after, protecting your baby is part of what it means to be a conscientious parent.

PART 2

Problems Along the Way

7 . The Baby Who Might Have Been: Early Pregnancy Loss

NAOMI COWAN HAD JUST BOUGHT her first maternity dress. She'd grinned as she looked in the mirror in the fitting room. For the first time she looked like a woman who was going to have a baby.

That afternoon Naomi noticed that she was spotting. By the time she got home from work she was bleeding more heavily and having menstruallike cramps. The pain intensified through the evening. When she called her doctor, Naomi was crying. "I knew I was losing the baby," she recalls. "And all I had to show for the whole experience was the new maternity dress. I felt that the pregnancy was over before it really began."

About 300,000 women—10 to 15 percent of all pregnant women— miscarry every year. In another 20,000 to 40,000 women, the fertilized egg cell implants itself somewhere other than in the uterus, resulting in an ectopic (out-of-place) pregnancy. More rarely, the fertilized egg degenerates and the placental tissue forms a mole that simulates the signs of normal pregnancy. Sometimes these events occur before a woman even realizes she is pregnant. More often early pregnancy losses occur just as the mother-to-be is adjusting to the prospect of having a baby. "You're left with nothing," says Naomi, "except your dreams of what might have been."

In this chapter we will explain why pregnancies fail and how each type of pregnancy loss is diagnosed and treated, discuss the outlook for future pregnancies, and describe the psychological impact of losing an unborn baby.

· Miscarriage

The medical term for a pregnancy that ends before the twentieth week of gestation is abortion, though most lay people use the word miscarriage to refer to a spontaneous abortion such as Naomi's. Approximately 95 percent of miscarriages occur before the sixteenth week; most by the eighth to tenth week. Miscarriages generally are chance occurrences that cannot be fully explained and that do not affect your ability to have a normal pregnancy and baby in the future. An estimated 70 to 90 percent of women who miscarry eventually become pregnant again.

Why Miscarriages Occur

In a classic scene in *Gone With The Wind*, Scarlett O'Hara loses her baby—and almost her life—after plunging down a long staircase. That is the sort of drama that movies are made of. In real life, most women who suffer falls and injuries do not miscarry. Cushioned by amniotic fluid, a baby is protected from all but the most severe types of trauma. Since the signs of a miscarriage often don't occur for several days or a week or two *after* the fetus dies, a loss rarely can be blamed on a fall or shock that happened a few hours before bleeding began.

In as many as one half to two thirds of miscarriages, the cause is a major genetic abnormality, usually a missing or extra chromosome (see Chapter 4). The embryo itself is defective and unable to develop normally. Nature seems to have its own mechanism for detecting devastating genetic flaws and ejecting the malformed embryo from the uterus.

The incidence of miscarriages also increases when the ovum is "old," that is, when fertilization occurs several days after the release of the egg cell from the ovary. In laboratory experiments, researchers have demonstrated that if fertilization occurs three days after the rise in body temperature that accompanies ovulation, pregnant animals are more likely to miscarry. It may be that the ovum had already begun to disintegrate at the time of fertilization. Doctors use the term "blighted ovum" to refer to an embryo that disintegrates or is absorbed by the surrounding tissue very early in pregnancy. Later, when the woman miscarries, the gestational sac expelled with the other products of pregnancy is empty.

Miscarriages occur more often in women who smoke, and the danger of a loss increases along with the number of cigarettes smoked. Certain drugs, including alcohol, also increase the likelihood of miscarriage. Women employed in certain occupations, such as dental hygiene, or married to men in certain fields, such as anesthesiology, have higher miscarriage rates than others.

Anatomy and medical history also play important roles. If you have a gynecologic anomaly, such as a double uterus, or numerous fibroid tumors (benign growths) in your uterus, you may be at greater risk. Exposure to diethylstilbestrol (DES) given to your mother before your birth may have altered your reproductive tract in ways that increase your risk of miscarrying. Two or more therapeutic abortions also may make you more susceptible. Midtrimester abortions—those performed from the fourth through sixth months—seem to pose a greater risk than earlier ones. It isn't clear exactly how an abortion affects a future pregnancy, but some physicians suspect that the problem is related to possible damage to the cervix or the uterine wall.

Deficiencies or disburbances within the womb can jeopardize a pregnancy. Some researchers have suggested that hormone imbalances, such as low levels of thyroid hormones or progesterone, may cause miscarriages. In general, no hormone supplements have been proven effective in preventing or decreasing the risk of miscarriage. Thyroid extracts have restored fertility to some hypothyroid women, but their impact on the risk of miscarriage is not clear.

Bacterial and viral infections, particularly those caused by T-mycoplasma microbes, have been implicated in some miscarriages, but the association is not well established. There is a definite increased risk in pregnant women who have a flare-up of systemic lupus erythematosus (SLE), an autoimmune disorder that affects the kidneys and blood vessels (see Chapter 15).

Surgery during pregnancy may increase the likelihood of miscarriage, depending on the site of the operation. The closer it is to the uterus, the greater is the danger of a loss. Some prenatal diagnostic tests, including amniocentesis and fetoscopy (see Chapter 5), pose a very slight risk of miscarriage.

Types of Miscarriage

Miscarriages occur for different reasons, and they do not produce the same symptoms or have the same implications for future pregnancies. If you have miscarried before, or if your risk is higher than usual, you should be aware of the various types of early pregnancy losses.

Threatened Miscarriage This term refers to a miscarriage that *may* happen but has not yet definitely occurred. Any bleeding in the first half of pregnancy can be a sign of a threatened miscarriage. However, early bleeding does *not* mean that you definitely will miscarry.

One of every four or five pregnant women bleeds or spots in the first months, particularly on the days when menstruation would normally occur. Fewer than half of these women eventually miscarry. The bleeding might be caused by polyps (growths in the cervix), other cervical lesions, or an IUD that was left in place. If the bleeding stops and you continue to gain weight and your baby continues to grow, the rest of your pregnancy should be normal.

Sometimes the bleeding persists, and neither you nor your obstetrician can be certain whether or not you've miscarried. Rather than take a wait-and-see approach, your doctor can perform certain tests to see if you're still pregnant. One is an analysis of your blood and urine to identify human chorionic gonadotropin (HCG), the hormone associated with pregnancy. If there are no trac s of HCG, you've definitely miscarried. But a positive test may not be definitive proof that you didn't miscarry, since HCG can remain in your body for several weeks after a fetus dies. The most precise test is an ultrasound scan, which reveals what is happening in the uterus. If the sonogram shows a living fetus, your chances of continuing the pregnancy are excellent despite the early bleeding.

In the past, various treatments for threatened miscarriages were tried. DES was one such drug, given to more than 25,000 women in the 1940s and 1950s to prevent a possible loss. More recently progestins, synthetic forms of progesterone, were used, but they too are hazardous to the developing baby and may only prolong or delay an eventual miscarriage. In rare incidences in which a woman has low progesterone levels *before* conception and in the first few months of pregnancy— before any sign of miscarriage—progesterone treatment may be helpful.

The current recommendation for a threatened miscarriage is restriction of activity and rest in bed. If the bleeding stops, you can get up in a day or two. If it persists and your doctor confirms that you miscarried in the first twelve weeks of pregnancy, he or she will perform a "D&C" (dilation and curettage), a procedure in which the cervix is opened and the contents of the uterus removed. If you miscarry in your second trimester, oxytocin, a hormone that induces contractions, or prostaglandins may be administered to complete the expulsion of the uterine contents. You should allow yourself ample time for rest and recovery afterward, and in order to prevent infection, you should not have intercourse while bleeding or for two weeks after the bleeding stops.

Inevitable Miscarriage The most typical sign of miscarriage is pain as well as bleeding. It may be cramplike at first and then intensify. A miscarriage is inevitable once your cervix dilates (opens) or the membranes of the amniotic sac break. Usually you feel a rush of fluid, followed by contractions of the uterus and expulsion of the gestational sac. You will be advised to stay in bed for at least forty-eight hours. If bleeding continues or you develop a fever, you may be hospitalized. A D&C may be performed, either in the hospital or in your doctor's office, to ensure that the uterus is completely emptied.

Incomplete Miscarriage In some miscarriages the fetus and placenta are not expelled completely. When the placenta, in whole or part, is retained in the uterus, bleeding—possibly quite heavy—continues. Obstetricians frequently use an aspiration, or low suction, device to remove the placental tissue, either in their offices or in an emergency room. Hospitalization is necessary if blood loss is severe.

Missed Miscarriage Sometimes the first trimester of a pregnancy is perfectly normal. Then the fetus dies, though the woman may or may not experience bleeding. Afterward, her uterus stops growing; her breasts become smaller; she may lose several pounds. However, the dead fetus remains in the uterus. As a rule, the products of the pregnancy are expelled eventually, as in an ordinary miscarriage. If this does not happen, the woman may develop serious blood abnormalities and may start to bleed from her nose, gums, or any sites of slight trauma. A D&C and hospitalization may be necessary.

Habitual Miscarriage A series of three or more miscarriages may be a chance occurrence or an indication of a hidden problem. There are two confirmed reasons for miscarriages to occur again and again: a genetic abnormality or a disorder of the uterus or cervix. You and your mate can find out more about your genetic makeup and potential problems from a genetic counselor (see Chapter 4). Your obstetrician may trace the problem to a uterine anomaly, such as a double, divided, or forked uterus, large fibroid tumors (myomas), or scarring within your uterus. Sometimes surgery can correct such problems before you become pregnant again.

Even when the cause of repeated miscarriages is not pinpointed, the "cure" rate is high: an estimated 70 to 85 percent of women who have had several losses eventually have normal pregnancies and healthy babies.

Incompetent Cervix This is a relatively rare problem in which the cervix painlessly opens in the second trimester, the amniotic membranes rupture, and a fetus too immature to survive is expelled. This sad sequence of events may repeat itself through several pregnancies. The cause is an "incompetent" cervix that can not resist the pressure of the growing gestational sac. This problem generally does not occur in women who have neither borne children before nor had cervical operations, nor does it happen before the sixteenth week, while the fetus and its sac are still relatively small.

There is a way of making an incompetent cervix competent. A suture, called a cerclage, is drawn tight around the cervix, leaving only a small opening. Just like the drawstring on a purse, it helps prevent the cervix from dilating (expanding). A cerclage usually is removed in the thirty-seventh week of pregnancy, and labor and delivery are allowed to proceed normally. Occasionally an obstetrician will sew up an incompetent cervix before pregnancy begins. The success rate is very high when the problem clearly is caused by an incompetent cervix. However, sometimes physicians use cerclages in the hope they will provide some benefit, even when it is not clear that an incompetent cervix is the cause of the miscarriages. In such circumstances, cerclages are much less likely to help.

Very rarely a woman may have a tear in her cervix so deep that it extends into her abdomen, or her cervix may be so short that a cerclage will not work. In the second trimester, her obstetrician can place sutures around the lower portion of the uterus to prevent a miscarriage. Because this operation is delicate and risky, the sutures usually are left in place if the woman wants other pregnancies. The babies are delivered by cesarean section.

· Ectopic Pregnancy

In an ectopic (out-of-place) pregnancy, a fertilized egg implants itself in the wrong place. Rather than developing within the uterus, the embryo begins to grow within the fallopian tube (the site of 95 percent of ectopic pregnancies) or in the abdomen, ovary, or cervix. A misplaced pregnancy rarely produces a healthy baby and can be a grave threat to the mother's life, particularly if the blood vessels of the gestational sac erode and cause a hemorrhage. Ectopic pregnancies are not uncommon: The estimates of their frequency range from 1 in every 84 to 1 in every 230 conceptions. The incidence has increased recently, possibly because pelvic infections, which add to the risk of ectopic pregnancy, have become more common.

Why Ectopic Pregnancy Occurs

The specific reasons why a fertilized egg is misguided are not clear, but the likelihood of an ectopic pregnancy increases in women with pelvic inflammatory disease (PID), or salpingitis. PID is the serious consequence of infections caused by IUDs or by sexually transmitted diseases. Because PID can scar and narrow the fallopian tubes, a fertilized egg may not make its way to the uterus. Usually both tubes are affected, and the damage, which can be severe, is irreversible.

An anatomical defect or adhesions of tissue inside the fallopian tubes also can interfere with the fertilized egg's journey to the uterus. Any surgery on the tubes, including attempts to open blocked tubes or to cut the tubes for sterilization, increases the likelihood of an ectopic pregnancy.

Diagnosis and Treatment

You may have an ectopic pregnancy and not suspect that you're pregnant at all, or you may believe that your pregnancy is absolutely normal. In the former instance, rather than menstruating, you may bleed slightly or spot. Your placenta will secrete human chorionic gonadotropin (HCG), the classic indicator of pregnancy, but in lower amounts, so a pregnancy test may or may not be positive.

You may not have any clue that something is wrong until you feel pain in your lower abdomen. It can be mild or very severe. Some women describe it as a sharp, tearing sensation. In some cases, the blood in the abdominal cavity irritates the diaphragm, so the neck and shoulders also are sore. Your abdomen will be tender to the touch. A vaginal exam may be quite painful, especially when the obstetrician touches or moves the cervix. If the tubal pregnancy has burst and internal bleeding is occurring, your pulse will be quite rapid and your blood pressure will fall. If you experience these symptoms, seek immediate care. The abdominal bleeding can lead to life-threatening shock.

In only about half of ectopic pregnancies can the obstetrician feel a mass in the pelvis simply by palpating your stomach. That's why, in the past, so many ectopic pregnancies were not detected before they burst. Today improved diagnostic techniques can identify a misplaced embryo before the danger to the mother intensifies.

The combination of a pregnancy test for HCG in your blood and urine and a sonogram gives the obstetrician the first clues. If the pregnancy test is positive but the ultrasound scan shows no evidence of a gestational sac in the uterus, your doctor will check for internal bleeding. The standard technique is culdocentesis, a method of sampling the fluid in a cul-de-sac, a cavity in the pelvis where blood would accumulate.

Once the diagnosis is made, treatment—surgical removal of the gestational sac, and frequently of the tube in which the embryo implanted itself—must be immediate to prevent further danger. Fifty percent of women who've had one ectopic pregnancy do become pregnant again; and 10 percent of them have another ectopic pregnancy. If one fallopian tube is badly scarred because of infection, the other tube is also likely to be scarred. Your obstetrician may try to salvage one tube if you want to conceive again, but your chances of having a normal pregnancy depend on the severity of the damage within the tubes. In one group of women in which the gestational sac was removed but the scarred tube preserved, 30 percent became pregnant again; 15 percent of these women had another ectopic pregnancy. If you do *not* want to become pregnant again, tubal sterilization can be performed quickly when the gestational sac is removed. This is not a reversible procedure.

· Molar Pregnancy

Occasionally a developing pregnancy degenerates and the placental tissue forms a grapelike structure called a hydatiform mole. This mole grows within the uterus, simulating the signs of normal pregnancy. Often a molar pregnancy isn't suspected until late in the first trimester or in the early midtrimester.

The primary symptom is bleeding, which ranges from spotting to hemorrhage. Frequently the uterus enlarges more rapidly than usual, exceeding the expected size for the gestational age of the fetus. No fetal heart action can be detected. Ultrasound is the best method of detecting a mole, because it produces characteristic patterns in response to sound waves.

A mole is removed by different methods, depending on its size and the woman's condition. These treatments include vacuum aspiration (suction), induction of contractions to expel the growth, or hysterectomy (removal of the uterus). Some moles are precancerous and lead to an increased risk of choriocarcinoma, a cancer of the reproductive organs; follow-up examinations are critically important to make sure cancer does not develop.

• Early Pregnancy Loss: A Private Tragedy

"It's just a miscarriage." "It was only an ectopic."

These are common reactions of the family and friends of couples who lose a baby early in pregnancy. But for the expectant parents, a miscarriage or ectopic pregnancy is the death of a dream. The baby they'd planned for and fantasized about will never arrive.

From an outsider's perspective, it may seem that parents can't become emotionally attached to a fetus they've never seen or felt. But a wanted baby, though faceless and formless within the womb, is very real. Its loss can be deeply painful.

Obviously, the circumstances of the pregnancy affect the parents' reaction. If the couple had a long history of infertility or no other children, they may be heartbroken when this hoped-for pregnancy ends. If the parents had not wanted this pregnancy at this time, they may feel sad but at the same time relieved.

Many women feel angry—at their doctor, their husbands (who may not seem to react as intensely to the loss), and themselves. Their emotions, like those of women who lose babies after delivery (see Chapter 22), must be acknowledged and expressed. Bottled up inside, these feelings can gnaw away at a woman's sense of self-esteem and her ability to function and enjoy life. It's not unusual for anger to turn inward into a lingering depression that troubles the woman, her partner, and their other children.

A third common by-product of a loss, along with anger and depression, is guilt. Even though nothing she did or didn't do caused the miscarriage or ectopic pregnancy a woman may blame herself. "I had a whole list of 'if only's,' " recalls one eagerly expectant mother who miscarried. "If only I hadn't gone skiing; if only we didn't have sex the night before; if only I didn't stay out so late last Saturday. . . . They went round and round in my head, until I felt absolutely miserable." Finally she admitted her "guilt" to her doctor. Within minutes, she learned that none of her activities could possibly have caused the miscarriage. "I could almost feel this terrible weight being lifted. For the first time, I could look at the baby's loss as a cruel twist of fate, not as a reflection of something I did."

The suddenness with which the symptoms of a miscarriage or ectopic pregnancy appear may stun a woman. After weeks of adjusting to pregnancy, it's all over. "I woke up one morning pregnant, healthy, and happy," recalls a woman who had an ectopic pregnancy. "Twelve hours later I was in a hospital emergency room, doubled over with pain, bleeding, and worried that I was going to lose this baby and my chance of ever having another baby."

It takes time for both body and mind to recover from such a blow. Both parents have to absorb what happened and come to terms with it. The immediate emotional turmoil gradually subsides but feelings of sadness or depression may surface again and again. The baby's due date may be an especially trying time, as well as the anniversary of the day of the miscarriage. Yet, like other wounds, this one too heals with time. The pain, as one counselor puts it, is "colored by the realization that life goes on in new forms and in new ways." And, for the majority of those who lose a baby early in pregnancy, the future holds the promise of another pregnancy, this time a successful one.

8 . *Little Babies: Growth Problems Before Birth*

HELPING BABIES WHO ARE SMALL for their gestational age (SGA) is one of the most difficult challenges in perinatology. About 30 to 40 percent of all infants that weigh less than 2,500 grams (5½ pounds) at birth are SGA babies; others are premature; others are both premature and SGA. For all these infants, starting off small can create very big problems. A baby that doesn't grow well in the womb is more likely to die before, during, or soon after birth, or to suffer serious illness or impairment.

One problem in treating SGA babies is diagnosing growth problems early enough to overcome them. Only a third of all serious growth impairments are detected before birth. Because early diagnosis can help save more babies' lives and prevent permanent damage, your obstetrician will keep a close eye on how your baby is growing. At various stages in your pregnancy, he or she will compare your baby's estimated size to an average weight for that stage, computed from data on thousands of pregnancies. Your baby will be classified as SGA if it weighs less than do 90 percent of babies of the same gestational age. In this chapter we will discuss the reasons why some babies have a growth problem, how it is diagnosed, and what you and your doctor can do to help a too-small baby.

· What Causes Growth Problems

In its nine months within your womb, your baby grows from a fertilized egg cell into a fully developed human being with 6,000 billion cells. This growth is anything but haphazard; normal fetal development follows an extraordinarily precise timetable and a predictable pattern. But sometimes something goes wrong, usually in the final trimester. The baby simply may stop growing, or its head will continue to grow but its body will not. A less frequent but more serious problem is a

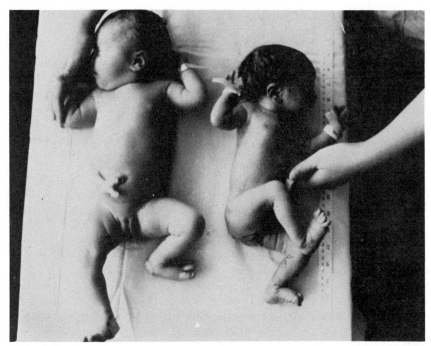

Both of these newborns spent just as much time in the womb, but the one on the right developed growth problems before birth

slowing of normal growth as early as the second trimester.

Why does a baby stop growing or slow down its growth rate in the womb? That's not an easy question to answer. If your baby seems smaller than it should be, your obstetrician will first consider some factors that might be influencing its size and that might not be problems at all. Heredity is one influence, since little women tend to have little babies, while large women have large babies. There also are differences among various racial and ethnic groups, so that a normal-sized baby for an Oriental woman may be smaller than a normal-sized baby for a Caucasian.

Usually a first baby will be smaller than his or her siblings. A second baby generally weighs about 130 grams (4½ ounces) more than its older brother or sister; a third baby will weigh even more, though the difference in size will not be as striking. The reasons why second- and third-born babies are bigger are not well understood, but it is possible that the blood vessels to the uterus, more developed after one pregnancy, become more efficient in nourishing the next baby. Sex also makes a difference in a baby's weight. At thirty-two weeks of gestation, male and female babies are about the same size, but by thirty-eight weeks, a male fetus weighs 150 to 200 grams (5–7 ounces) more than a female.

The father's size does not have much impact on how much a baby weighs at birth, although his height will be a major influence on how tall the child eventually will be.

In other circumstances, a baby will be smaller than it could and should be because of an impairment of normal growth. This is more likely to happen if the mother is under 18—possibly because teenagers have greater nutritional needs themselves and often don't eat a well-balanced diet—or if she is over 35. Older women are more likely to have hypertension or other medical problems that affect the blood vessels and, therefore, the supply of nutrients to a growing baby. If your sister has had an SGA baby, you're likely to have one too, regardless of your age; and having one SGA baby increases the probability of the next child also being small.

A key factor in any baby's birth weight is the nourishment it receives in the womb. During pregnancy your body is synthesizing new tissues more rapidly than at any other time in your life, and good nutrition is essential for your health and your baby's development. As we said in Chapter 3, you should gain at least 24 to 27 pounds. If you gain less than 20 pounds, you are much more likely to have an SGA baby. The quality of the foods you eat is as significant as the quantity of weight you gain. Be sure to include foods from the five basic food groups— proteins, milk products, vegetables and fruits rich in vitamin C, grains, and other vegetables and fruits—in your daily diet.

Sometimes the problem is not in what or how much you eat, but in making sure that the nutrients reach your baby. During pregnancy your blood vessels carry oxygen and food to your baby. Anything that interferes with the flow of blood to the uterus and placenta can impede your baby's growth. The most common complication associated with impaired blood flow is hypertension (high blood pressure), and problems related to this condition are responsible for at least 20 to 30 percent of prenatal growth impairments. Other diseases that affect the blood vessels, including kidney and vascular disorders, also can slow the rate of normal growth in the womb. Proper treatment for these disorders is essential for your sake and your baby's. Lack of oxygen, which may occur at altitudes higher than 10,000 feet, can interfere with a baby's growth by decreasing the amount of oxygen in the mother's bloodstream.

A frequent—and preventable—cause of growth impairment is cigarette smoking. The baby of a mother who smokes heavily throughout pregnancy may weigh 150 grams (5 ounces) less than it should. The more cigarettes the mother smokes, the less oxygen the baby receives— and the less it grows. Alcohol and hard drugs also interfere with normal growth; the babies of alcoholics and heroin addicts often suffer severe growth retardation.

Some growth problems have more to do with the babies themselves than with their mothers. For example, if two or more babies are competing for the available supply of nutrients, they're likely to have lower birth weights than babies who don't have to share food before birth. If you are expecting twins or triplets, good nutrition will be all-important. As you will see in Chapter 18, your weight gain may be half again the normal 24–27 pounds because you need to provide significantly more than the usual amount of proteins, carbohydrates, folic acid, vitamins, and iron.

The average birth weight for 40 to 60 percent of all twins is less than 2,500 grams (5½ pounds). Identical twins tend to be smaller than fraternal ones; those sharing a placenta and gestational sac are at greatest risk of growth impairment. Occasionally one of the babies will get a much larger share of the food supply. This causes problems for both. The smaller twin may develop the same complications as other babies with severe growth retardation. The larger twin, with an abnormally high blood volume and low blood pressure, may develop heart failure and potentially fatal circulation disorders.

Sometimes an abnormality of the placenta or umbilical cord causes a growth problem. Because the umbilical cord is your baby's lifeline and because the placenta is the primary source of nourishment in the womb, such disorders can have a serious impact on how your baby grows. The placenta typically matures, or ages, through the course of pregnancy. If your baby remains in the womb for more than forty weeks, the "old" placenta may not continue to provide adequate nourishment. As a result, your baby may stop gaining weight and actually begin to lose weight; this is part of a problem referred to as "postmaturity" (see Chapter 17).

In 10 to 20 percent of SGA babies, a congenital malformation, chromosomal defect, or serious prenatal infection is the cause of the growth problem. The two infections that pose the greatest danger to normal growth are rubella (German measles) and cytomegalovirus, the most common prenatal infection (see Chapter 16).

• Diagnosing a Growth Problem

Your obstetrician will keep track of your baby's development from your first prenatal visit until delivery. One of the reasons that you are asked the date of the first day of your last menstrual period is so your doctor can estimate your baby's age and whether its size is appropriate. (The methods of dating a pregnancy are described in Chapter 3.) Throughout pregnancy, your weight gain and fundal height are indicators of how well your baby is growing. If they seem higher or lower than usual, your obstetrician may use ultrasound to follow your baby's growth. Repeated every few weeks, sonograms can show whether your baby's total body growth is lagging, whether the diameter of its head is smaller than usual, or whether the growth of both body and head is impaired. Sometimes ultrasound can identify the cause of the growth problem, such as a multiple pregnancy or an anomaly.

SGA babies are not as strong as others because they don't get adequate oxygen and nourishment. For these frail babies, the womb often becomes an increasingly hazardous environment, and they face a greater chance of death in the last weeks of gestation. To prevent a stillbirth, your doctor will evaluate your baby's condition frequently in the last trimester. The standard tests of fetal well-being, described in Chapter 5, include nonstress and stress testing. Measurements of estriol levels in urine tend to be abnormally low in 70 to 90 percent of SGA babies and normal in 10 to 30 percent, so the results are not clear-cut. You can monitor your baby's well-being by counting its movements every day and notifying your doctor if there is a marked decrease or cessation of activity.

If your baby is in danger, early delivery may be the best option. Very often the stress of life in the womb speeds up the lung maturation process, so SGA babies are less likely to develop respiratory problems after birth. Because it can be very difficult to get a clear picture of an SGA baby's condition, your obstetrician may ultimately rely on clinical judgment and experience in timing the delivery.

· What to Expect

If your baby is having growth problems, you can help. The final months of pregnancy are the time of most rapid development, when a baby normally can gain an ounce a day. Eat nutritiously and avoid cigarettes and alcohol, since they can interfere with blood flow to the uterus. You also might spend more time lying on your side in bed; this enhances the flow of blood to your baby.

You should anticipate frequent monitoring of your baby in the last months of pregnancy. Because of the increased risk of problems before, during, and after birth, your doctor may transfer you to a hospital with special facilities for evaluating your baby before and during birth and for treating any problems after birth. SGA babies fare much better as newborns if transferred to a perinatal center while still within the womb.

SGA babies tend to be much more vulnerable to the stresses of being born. During normal labor, a baby's oxygen supply is cut off briefly during a contraction. Usually this is not dangerous. However, the risk of damage or death because of oxygen deprivation (a condition called hypoxia) is compounded for SGA babies because the placenta may not be providing adequate oxygen and blood in the periods between as well as during contractions. An electronic fetal monitor (see page 52) can detect worrisome abnormalities in the baby's heart rate. If necessary, fetal scalp sampling (see page 55) will be used to get a better idea of how the baby is withstanding the stress of labor. If there are danger signs, a cesarean delivery may be performed to avoid the rigors of a vaginal delivery. Whether a baby is born vaginally or by a cesarean, a specialist in newborn care may be in the delivery room to help it take its first breaths. SGA babies are more likely to release meconium (sterile waste) into the amniotic fluid. If they have swallowed or inhaled any meconium, the doctor will begin suctioning the nose and throat as soon as the head emerges. When completely delivered, the baby will be taken to a special heated table in or near the delivery room. The doctor will clear the airway and vocal cords of meconium and if necessary, provide mechanical assistance in breathing. A blood sample is tested for signs of polycythemia, an excess of red blood cells that sometimes causes "sludging" and interferes with normal circulation.

SGA babies have different problems in their first days than babies who were born too soon. They are less likely to develop respiratory distress, but they may have lung infections or hemorrhages. Low levels of sugar (hypoglycemia) and of calcium (hypocalcemia) are common problems; they are easily corrected but can create serious dangers if not detected and treated. Sometimes the cause of growth impairment in the womb can mean more problems after birth. Fetal alcohol syndrome, for example, can interfere with prenatal development *and* cause lifelong mental and physical abnormalities. Some genetic defects or maternal prenatal infections also may increase the risks to a baby's survival and its normal development.

· Prognosis

Your baby's birth weight affects its chances for survival, its health in the first days of life, and its long-term physical and intellectual ability. Generally the smaller the baby is, the bigger the problems it will face as a child and as an adult. Some SGA babies develop subtle disorders, such as learning disabilities, that show up years after their birth and that may be related to difficulties in the womb or in the process of being born. However, most SGA babies who receive proper care during pregnancy, birth, and the first weeks of life do very well in the long term. Eventually they catch up in size to other children their age. Their IQs are normal, and they have no abnormalities in behavior or movement.

9 . *Premature Babies: Buying Time in the Womb*

APPROXIMATELY 10 percent of all babies—some 300,000 each year—are born too soon. They are among the most vulnerable of newborns. Thrust into the world before they are ready to survive on their own, they account for 75 percent of perinatal deaths not associated with genetic defects and for 50 percent of neurologic handicaps in infants. Obstetricians and pediatricians consider prematurity the biggest clinical problem they face. In many ways, it also is the most perplexing.

Preterm labor is defined as the onset of rhythmic contractions of the uterus after the twentieth and before the thirty-seventh week of pregnancy, resulting in the thinning (effacement) and opening (dilation) of the cervix. Why does nature's timetable for labor occasionally go awry? Why are some babies forced from the womb weeks or even months before their time? Despite years of research, there still are no clear answers.

Even though medical understanding of the causes of preterm labor remains limited, there is new hope for babies at risk of being born too soon. In the 1970s neonatologists refined the techniques and technology that have helped save thousands of "preemies." In the 1980s the emphasis has shifted to preventing too-early deliveries rather than dealing with their consequences. It may be possible to delay as many as 50 percent of all preterm births—if more pregnant women learn the warning signals of premature labor and seek immediate treatment. In this chapter we will describe the risk factors for preterm labor, its early signs, and the ways in which you and your doctor can assure your baby of the time it needs to prepare for a healthy life.

· Recognizing the Risks

Realizing that you are at risk is the first step in overcoming the dangers of preterm labor. Many obstetricians evaluate the likelihood of too-early labor at the first prenatal visit. Some assign a different numerical value to various risk factors. However, current risk-rating systems identify only about half the women who eventually go into preterm labor. That's why every pregnant woman should be aware of the risk factors and the warning signs.

Medical conditions, socioeconomic stresses, daily habits, and complications in your current pregnancy can add to the probability of preterm labor. The most significant risk factor is premature labor or birth in a previous pregnancy. If you've ever started labor too early, there is a 25 to 50 percent likelihood that you will do so again. You're also at greater risk if you've had two or more miscarriages or abortions (especially in the midtrimester), if you were exposed to DES (diethylstilbestrol) before your birth, if you've had biopsies (tissue sampling) that involved dilation of your cervix, if you have a uterine anomaly, or if you've had repeated kidney or urinary tract infections.

Your risk also increases if you're under 18 or over 35, if you're less than 5 feet tall, or if you weigh less than 100 pounds. If your husband is unemployed, if you're a single parent, or if you have two or more preschool children at home, the physical, psychological, and financial pressures can make preterm labor more likely. Smoking more than ten cigarettes a day multiplies the odds. A long, tiring commute of more than an hour and a half every day or very strenuous work, particularly if it involves continuous standing, physical effort, or tension, may also increase the risks.

A woman expecting twins or triplets is much more likely to begin labor early; half of all twin pregnancies culminate in premature delivery. Among the other pregnancy complications that add to the likelihood of preterm labor are: abdominal surgery during pregnancy; hydramnios (an excess of amniotic fluid); placenta previa (a disorder in which the placenta is located at the bottom of the womb, covering the cervix); opening or thinning of your cervix; bleeding after your twelfth week; uterine irritability; engagement of your baby's head as early as the thirty-second or thirty-fourth week; fever; a weight loss of more than 5 pounds; a weight gain of less than 12 pounds by your thirty-second week; fibroid tumors; hypertension; and bacteriuria (bacteria in a urine sample, a sign of infection). If any of these conditions occur, discuss them with your obstetrician. Not all are equally serious, but certain risk factors or combinations of factors significantly increase the chance that your baby will be born too soon.

· Detecting the Warning Signals

Very often preterm labor begins so insidiously that you may not be aware of what's happening until it's too late to stop the contractions. You may develop only one symptom or several. The important thing is to notify your doctor of what's happening rather than wait and see what happens next. The most common signals of preterm labor are: a dull, low backache; a feeling of tightness or a dragging sensation in your abdomen, somewhat similar to menstrual cramping; a sense of

Detecting "Silent" Preterm Contractions

1. While lying in bed or on the sofa, place your *fingertips* on the top of your uterus.

2. Contractions usually begin at the top of your uterus. They are best described as a "tension" or "hardening" of your uterus, similar to what the tip of your nose feels like or harder. If your uterus is contracting, you will actually feel your abdomen get "tight" or "hard" and then relax (soften). You may even see it "move up" slightly in your abdomen. The tightness will increase, reaching a peak, and then slowly decrease.

3. If your uterus is tightening and relaxing, be sure to note the time each contraction starts, how long it lasts, and how often these "tightenings" are occurring. Time the contractions for an hour.

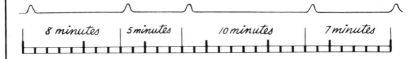

TIME UTERINE CONTRACTIONS FROM THE BEGINNING OF ONE
CONTRACTION TO THE BEGINNING OF THE NEXT CONTRACTION.

4. If you are experiencing uterine contractions at regular intervals, and any of the other warning signs and symptoms of premature labor, *call your doctor, clinic, or delivery room. Do not wait for the symptoms to disappear.* They may not disappear, and your baby may be born too early.

Sometimes "silent" contractions can occur *without any* warning signs and symptoms. Therefore, it is important for any pregnant woman to feel her uterus for contractions at least twice a day for half-hour periods. It is also helpful to palpate (feel) for contractions at the same time each day, because sometimes women will experience contractions in the morning and not in the evening, or in the afternoon and not in the evening.

If you find that you are experiencing regular contractions—that is, every 10–15 minutes or closer for an hour—*notify your doctor, clinic, or delivery room.*

pressure on your lower abdomen, back, or thighs; and intestinal cramps, sometimes with diarrhea. The regular premature tightening and relaxation of your uterine muscles are painless, but you can detect "silent" contractions with your fingertips, as described in the box on page 90. If they occur at intervals of less than ten minutes and continue for more than an hour, seek immediate medical care. Sometimes you may have some or all of these symptoms, yet an examination will show no cervical changes. Conversely, your cervix may begin to change without any external symptoms. If you are at high risk of preterm labor, your cervix can be checked for signs of dilation or effacement every week or two from the twentieth week of pregnancy until term.

· What to Expect

Bed rest is the cornerstone of treatment for preterm labor. If you develop the early signs, your obstetrician may recommend that you spend several extra hours a day in bed, preferably on your side. You may have to restrict your physical activity. That means no exercise, no sustained lifting (whether it's of laundry baskets, groceries, or children), no heavy cleaning, and no taxing work outside or inside the house. Because anxiety can increase the chance of preterm labor, you should try to avoid stress as much as you can. Often it helps to talk over your concerns—about yourself, your baby, your family, or whatever—with your partner, a friend, or your doctor.

Weekly or biweekly checkups are essential for monitoring cervical changes. These may be the only trips you're allowed to make outside your home. You also may have to limit or restrict sexual activity, because orgasm and the release of prostaglandins from the sperm and cervix during intercourse may irritate the uterus and cause cervical softening in some women. You usually can continue childbirth classes and practice the breathing exercises, but you shouldn't participate in the more rigorous workouts. You also should not begin preparation of your breast for nursing, since this may release oxytocin, a hormone that stimulates contractions.

If you experience regular, persistent contractions, you will be examined and, if your cervix is opening or thinning, hospitalized. An electronic fetal monitor placed around your abdomen will record the duration and frequency of contractions and the baby's heart beats. Your urine will be analyzed for signs of bacterial infection, which may have caused the preterm contractions. You should expect frequent vaginal exams to check on cervical changes. Occasionally the hospital bed is put in what is called the Trendelenburg position, so your head is lower than your feet and pressure is taken off your cervix. If contractions continue, you may be given medication to relax your uterus. The agents currently used belong to a class of drugs called the beta-adrenergics; their brand names include Ritodrine, Vasodilan, Partusisten, Albuteral, and Bricanyl. They inhibit contractions by causing chemical changes in the cells of the uterus and are most effective if administered before the cervix has thinned out and opened to 3 or 4 centimeters, and before the amniotic membranes rupture.

Initially these drugs are given intravenously, either for a minimum of twenty-four hours or until contractions stop. While you are on IV therapy, you cannot sit up or leave your bed. You may experience various side effects, including a slight decrease in blood pressure, an increase in your pulse rate, palpitations of your heart, tremors, nausea, light-headedness, nasal congestion, flushing, or a feeling of warmth. The most serious complication, which is very rare, is pulmonary edema, a buildup of fluid in the lungs; if this develops, the labor-inhibiting drugs must be stopped.

Serious side effects occur most frequently with high doses. Once your contractions are under control, you will be switched to intramuscular injections or oral doses every two to four hours. You may continue taking labor-inhibiting drugs until your thirty-seventh week, when the danger of a preterm birth is past. Most women are able to return home after a few days of IV and oral treatment in the hospital, although they have to restrict their physical activities and spend at least part of the time on bed rest.

Other approaches have been used to contain preterm labor, including intravenous doses of ethanol (alcohol), which causes all the unpleasant side effects of drunkenness, and magnesium sulfate, a drug more frequently administered to prevent seizures in women with preeclampsia (page 105). Drugs (such as aspirin) that block the synthesis of prostaglandins—chemicals that play a role in inducing labor—may be effective, but since large doses of these agents can create risks to the baby that outweigh the potential benefits, they are not considered safe for use.

Sometimes, despite all efforts, delivery cannot be delayed for more than a few days. Your cervix may have opened to a width of more than 3 or 4 centimeters or may have completely thinned out. If this happens before the twenty-ninth week of pregnancy, the baby has only a fifty-fifty chance of survival. You may be transferred to a hospital with a specially staffed and equipped intensive-care nursery so these services will be available to help your baby from the moment of birth.

Your obstetrician may attempt to prevent some dangers to your baby in its first days in the world, primarily respiratory distress syndrome, a potentially fatal breathing disorder. This problem occurs most often in premature babies whose lungs have not yet produced a crucial substance called surfactant, which keeps the tiny air sacs inflated. You may be given two injections of a cortisonelike drug, such as betamethasone, to speed up production of surfactant. This powerful agent can help to save your baby's life by greatly decreasing the risk of respiratory distress after birth. But it has been in use for only a few years, so its long-term safety has not yet been established.

· Premature Rupture of the Membranes

A sudden gush of fluid from your vagina means that the membranes of your amniotic sac have broken. In most pregnancies they do not rupture until labor begins. The potential risk to your baby depends on when the membranes break. If you are less than thirty-two weeks pregnant, most obstetricians take a wait-and-see approach because of the extreme prematurity of the baby. Its chances for survival will improve considerably if delivery can be postponed for just a few weeks. If you are between the thirty-second and thirty-seventh weeks, the primary worry is the increased likelihood of an infection that could threaten the baby's survival. Your doctor may perform an amniocentesis to see whether your baby's lungs are mature; if they are, he or she may induce labor or perform a cesarean delivery. Your doctor will monitor you closely for any signs of infection and may induce labor if infection becomes a threat.

· Preterm Delivery

Sometimes a baby is born early because of circumstances beyond medical control. In other instances, a delivery is deliberately scheduled before term because the baby will be safer out in the world than in the womb. This occurs most frequently in pregnancies complicated by blood pressure problems, diabetes, and other medical disorders. The deliberate decision to deliver a baby early usually is based on tests that monitor its condition in the womb and that evaluate its lung maturity.

Whether a preterm delivery occurs in spite of or because of medical intervention, your baby will be monitored very carefully throughout the process. A premature baby, smaller than others and more fragile, is more vulnerable to the stresses of labor. Electronic fetal monitoring indicates how well it is withstanding the rigorous process of being born; if there are signs of fetal distress, a cesarean delivery may be performed.

· Prognosis

Almost all premature babies require some special care. If they are not delivered at hospitals with intensive-care nurseries, they may be transferred to the nearest such center. In many ways these newborns are more like fetuses than small versions of full-term infants. Downy hair still covers their bodies; their skin is often as transparent and fragile as parchment; their arms and legs are as thin as matchsticks.

The differences go beyond appearances: Because their lungs may not yet have manufactured surfactant to keep the tiny air sacs (alveoli) open, they are at great risk of developing respiratory distress. In 1970, 70 percent of preemies with this disorder died; today the mortality rate is less than 20 percent, in part because of advances in prenatal treatment and in part because of therapy after delivery. Among the improved methods of helping premature babies breathe is a system called CPAP—for "continuous positive airway pressure"—that keeps the alveoli open by means of a constant supply of pressurized oxygen, administered through a tube in the windpipe.

Preemies are prone to a host of other serious problems. Their temperatures can fall suddenly, creating acute physiological stress. Their levels of blood sugar (essential for brain functioning) or calcium (critical for muscle functioning) may drop and need immediate correction. About 40 percent of those weighing less than 1,500 grams at birth develop "bleeds," hemorrhages within the skull that range from minor leaks in the fluid-filled ventricles of the brain to massive bleeding that causes permanent brain damage. Occasionally another problem starts a few weeks after delivery, usually when most premature babies seem to be improving: necrotizing enterocolitis (NEC). For reasons that are not well understood, the delicate lining of the intestines is sloughed off, predisposing the baby to infection by its own bacteria. On constant guard against this threat, the nurses and doctors may check a baby's abdominal size and bowel movements several times a day. Their greatest fear is that the bowel will rupture, spilling its contents into the abdomen. Occasionally part of the intestine has to be removed.

Yet despite these hazards, alarming though they may sound, the prognosis for premature babies is better than ever: At many perinatal centers, 80 to 85 percent of those infants that weigh 1,000 to 1,250 grams (2¼ to 2½ pounds) at birth and 60 to 70 percent of those that weigh less than 1,000 grams are overcoming the perils of their too-early entry into the world. Various studies back up these statistical reports, confirming that the majority of preemies grow up to be normal and healthy—intellectually and physically.

10 . Vulnerable Babies: Rh and Other Blood Incompatibility Problems

SHERRI DALTON'S BULGING BELLY, stained with a yellowish antiseptic solution, gleams with a golden hue against the dark green surgical drapes covering the rest of her body. A radiologist presses a device that produces high-frequency sound waves against her glistening skin. As the ultrasonic echoes are transformed into black-and-white images, all the eyes in the examining room focus on a small television-type screen. Staring intently at the viewer, the obstetrician pushes a long thin needle through Sherri's skin into the abdominal cavity of her 29-week-old baby. Working quickly, he injects carefully measured amounts of packed red blood cells. Each time he pushes the syringe, the blood released inside the fetus forms a swirl of bubbles on the sonogram screen. Sherri cranes her neck to watch, biting her lip anxiously. "Poor little thing," she murmurs, "my poor little baby."

Sherri, like 12 percent of all Americans, does not have a substance in her blood called the Rh factor; her baby does. In response to this incompatibility, protective antibodies from her blood are crossing the placenta to attack and destroy the red blood cells of her unborn baby. Without a supply of healthy blood cells, her baby might not survive.

Twenty years ago the notion of a blood transfusion before birth seemed revolutionary. Today this therapy for the unborn is routine, although so much progress has been made in stopping Rh problems before they start that fewer babies need intrauterine transfusions. In this chapter we will describe the conquest of Rh disease, and explain what causes Rh and other blood incompatibility problems and how they can be prevented and treated.

· What Causes Rh Incompatibility

"Rh" refers to a group of substances in blood first identified in experiments with rhesus monkeys. While there are several Rh factors, the

Rh positive father

Rh negative mother

During Pregnancy

Rh negative mother with Rh positive baby

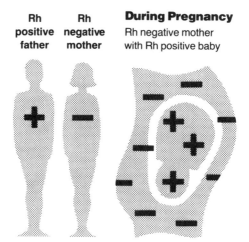

At Delivery

Rh positive baby's blood cells enter mother's bloodstream

Invading Rh positive blood cells cause the production of Rh antibodies

Months Later

Rh antibodies remain in mother's bloodstream

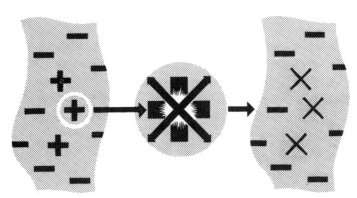

Subsequent Pregnancy

The Rh antibodies attack the baby's blood cells causing Rh disease

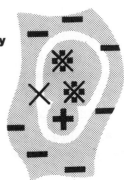

most significant is Rh_D. About 85 percent of American whites and 94 percent of blacks have this factor in their blood and are called Rh-positive; those who do not have it are Rh-negative. The presence or absence of the Rh factor has no impact on health. The only potential danger occurs when an Rh-positive man and an Rh-negative woman conceive a baby. Not all their children will be vulnerable, because not all of them will be Rh-positive. If the father has both an Rh-positive and an Rh-negative gene, there is a 50 percent chance that he will pass on the Rh-positive gene. If he does, there is no danger unless the Rh-negative mother has been "sensitized." This means that her blood has mingled with blood containing the Rh factor and, in response, her body has produced antibodies to destroy this foreign substance. (An antibody is a protein, manufactured by the body's protective immune system, that reacts specifically against the foreign body—in this case, the Rh-positive cells—that triggered its production.)

If you are Rh-negative, you are not likely to encounter any problems the first time you conceive an Rh-positive baby, because the blood of a mother and her unborn baby rarely mix until the pregnancy ends. Only 1½ to 2 percent of Rh-negative women become sensitized during pregnancy, most after 28 weeks. However, during an abortion, miscarriage, or delivery, there is a 10 to 15 percent chance that fetal blood cells will enter your bloodstream, triggering the production of Rh antibodies. Because of the variability in the way that Rh-negative individuals react to Rh-positive blood, you may not be sensitized even if your blood mingles with a fairly large amount of your baby's—or your body's defensive system may react to just a teaspoonful of its blood. If this occurs and you conceive another Rh-positive baby thereafter, your antibodies will spring into action, crossing the placenta to destroy the Rh-containing blood cells in the fetus in a process called hemolysis. Your unborn baby will produce more and more red blood cells (a condition called erythroblastosis fetalis), but it still may not be able to maintain an adequate supply of blood, particularly as it gets bigger. Because of this deficiency in healthy blood cells, the baby's body may become swollen; this can occur before or after birth, and is called hydrops. Pockets of fluid called ascites may form within its abdomen. Its heart, struggling to pump blood through its body and the placenta, may be unable to function properly. If not treated, these problems can be fatal or can cause severe brain damage.

• Preventing Rh Problems

In 1968 medical scientists discovered a way to prevent Rh-incompatibility problems. They noted that Rh-negative women who had been sensitized to Rh-positive blood had a high concentration of Rh antibodies in their gamma globulin, a blood component of the body's immune

RhoGAM is administered to Rh negative mother within 72 hours of delivery or miscarriage

RhoGAM prevents the formation of Rh antibodies

Mother's bloodstream does not contain Rh antibodies

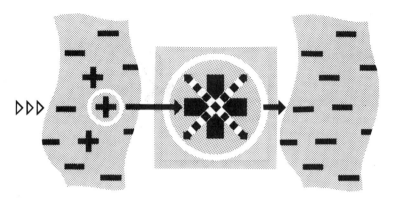

Baby develops normally. RhoGAM should again be administered following delivery or miscarriage to continue protection.

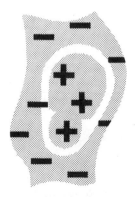

system. What would happen if their gamma globulin was injected into the blood of an Rh-negative woman at the time she was exposed to Rh-positive blood cells? Would the borrowed antibodies attack the Rh-positive cells from the fetus before the mother's immune system began to take action? As they demonstrated, that is exactly what does occur. When injected into the mother's bloodstream, the borrowed antibodies quickly coat and destroy the foreign fetal blood cells in the mother's circulation. The mother's body never manufactures any Rh antibodies, thus preventing Rh sensitization, and there is no threat of damage to any future children. But the key to the success of this approach is timing: The mother has to have the injections at the time when fetal blood cells are most likely to mingle with her blood—that means immediately after every delivery, miscarriage, or abortion.

The substance containing the anti-Rh antibodies is most commonly referred to as RhoGAM, although there are other brand names, such as Gamulin and HypRho-D. It is 98 to 99 percent effective in preventing the production of Rh antibodies; for unknown reasons, it fails to protect a small percentage of recipients. RhoGAM should be administered after delivery, miscarriage, or abortion to every woman at risk of becoming sensitized. Some obstetricians recommend RhoGAM at 28 weeks, as well as after delivery, in all Rh-negative women, whether or not they show any evidence of sensitization. This reduces the number of women who become sensitized before delivery from 1½ or 2 percent to less than .5 percent. However, this approach is not uniformly accepted. Antenatal RhoGAM is advised if there is abnormal bleeding during pregnancy and when amniocentesis or fetoscopy is performed.

• Treating Rh Disease

At your first prenatal visit, your obstetrician will test your blood to see if you're Rh-negative and if you've been sensitized to the Rh factor. If you're Rh-negative and *not* sensitized, your blood will be checked periodically throughout pregnancy to make sure no Rh antibodies have been manufactured. You will be given RhoGAM after delivery.

If you have become sensitized, you will be monitored closely. In the first pregnancy after sensitization, the level of Rh antibodies in your blood may rise steadily, indicating increasing danger to the Rh-positive baby. Once the antibodies reach a certain level, your obstetrician will need more information than a blood test can provide. He or she will perform an amniocentesis, a sampling of the amniotic fluid, to evaluate the baby's condition. The sample of the fluid is analyzed for evidence of bilirubin, the yellowish pigment released in the destruction of red blood cells. The color and density of the fluid indicate the severity of the damage caused by the Rh antibodies and the degree of anemia (red blood cell deficiency) in your baby. As we mentioned before, you may receive RhoGAM at 28 weeks or if you undergo amniocentesis or have abnormal bleeding.

If the baby is in jeopardy, an intrauterine transfusion provides it with the blood cells it needs to prevent permanent damage or death in the womb. This procedure, first performed in the mid-1960s, has increased by 50 percent the number of babies with Rh incompatibility who survive pregnancy and develop normally. There is a 5 to 10 percent risk of a miscarriage during each intrauterine transfusion, as well as a risk of premature rupture of the membranes, preterm labor, infection, or puncture of a blood vessel. However, these transfusions have become significantly safer and easier with the use of ultrasound to pinpoint the location of the fetal abdominal cavity.

The success of intrauterine transfusions depends on how much damage the antibodies have caused early in your pregnancy. If a transfusion is needed by the twenty-third week, the prognosis is poor, and there may be no more than a 15 percent chance for the baby's survival. If a transfusion isn't required until the thirtieth week, there is about an 85 percent chance of survival. Because the antibodies continue to destroy red blood cells throughout the rest of the pregnancy, the baby will need additional fresh cells, and transfusions will be repeated every ten to fourteen days. By the thirty-second week, the risk of an early delivery may be less than the danger involved in another transfusion. The obstetrician will rely on the results of the various tests of fetal well-being and of lung maturity in scheduling delivery. If your cervix is "unripe"—that is, if it hasn't begun to soften and thin out—it may not be possible to induce labor. If labor is prolonged and difficult, the stress of vaginal delivery may jeopardize a baby who's already developed medical complications because of Rh incompatibility. In both of these circumstances, a cesarean delivery will be performed to minimize the risks to the baby.

If bilirubin has built up in the baby's body, immediate care after birth is essential to prevent severe brain damage. You probably will be transferred before labor to a hospital with special facilities for sick newborns. At delivery, a specialist in infant care will stand by with a supply of fresh blood cells and equipment for an immediate transfusion. If necessary, the baby's blood, which contains immature red cells, dangerous amounts of bilirubin, and destructive Rh antibodies, will be drawn out and replaced with equal amounts of Rh-negative blood; this is called an exchange transfusion. A baby may require a single transfusion or five or more transfusions in the first week of its life.

· Other Blood Incompatibility Problems

As the threat of Rh disease has eased, more attention has focused on pregnancies complicated by other blood incompatibilities. RhoGAM is effective only in preventing a reaction to Rh_D; it does not have an effect on the so-called irregular antibodies, which also can be a threat to an unborn or newborn baby.

In theory almost every pregnancy could be complicated by the fact that a baby is likely to inherit some blood component from its father that is not in its mother's blood. In actuality, very few women produce antibodies against these foreign blood components. The most common blood incompatibility problem other than Rh involves mothers with Type O blood and babies with Type A or B blood. The mother may produce antibodies that destroy the baby's blood cells and release bilirubin into its bloodstream.

Most pregnant women are screened for potential ABO problems at the same time that their blood is tested for Rh factor. Unlike Rh disease, ABO incompatibility rarely threatens the life of the baby before birth. It can occur in a first pregnancy and is likely, but not certain, to recur in subsequent pregnancies. It is more common in blacks than whites and affects about 20 percent of newborns, although only 5 percent of these babies—1 percent of all infants—ever develop any overt problems. The most frequent consequence is hyperbilirubinemia, which causes jaundice. A baby with a high bilirubin level is treated with phototherapy (exposure to light, which breaks down the bilirubin); an exchange transfusion is rarely needed.

· Prognosis

The prognosis for newborns with Rh disease depends on what happened before birth. If their blood supply in the womb was inadequate and pockets of fluid formed in the abdomen, the babies are likely to suffer complications. If the blood supply before birth was adequate, they have an excellent chance of complete recovery. In one review of fifteen follow-up studies of babies with Rh problems, researchers found that most were developing normally at periods from one month to ten years after birth. The overwhelming majority of babies who had received intrauterine transfusions before birth had no physical or neurological problems as newborns or children. Babies with other blood incompatibility problems also did well if treated promptly in the days after their birth.

The brightest hope for Rh-related disorders is not in treatment, but in prevention. If RhoGAM were given to every Rh-negative woman every time there is a risk of sensitization, few Rh-positive babies would be at risk or would require special treatment before and after birth. Someday a similar form of prevention may be available to protect babies from other blood incompatibilities.

11 . *Problems Related to High Blood Pressure (Hypertension)*

BLOOD PRESSURE is a term that most of us are familiar with, but a concept that few of us understand. It is created by the contractions of the heart muscle, which pumps blood through your body, and the resistance of the walls of the vessels through which the blood flows. Each time your heart beats, your blood pressure goes up and down within a limited range. It is highest when the heart contracts; this is called systolic blood pressure. It is lowest between contractions; that is diastolic blood pressure. A blood pressure reading consists of the systolic measurement over the diastolic measurement, recorded in millimeters of mercury (mmHg). A normal nonpregnant woman for example, might have a reading of 120/80.

If your arteries squeeze down too hard on the blood flowing through them, you will have high blood pressure, or hypertension. This silent, symptom-free problem affects 26 million Americans. Its causes are unknown, although certain factors such as obesity, genetic predisposition (as indicated by family history), and smoking increase the risk. Some cases of hypertension are the result of medical problems that affect the blood vessels, such as kidney disease or diabetes.

Disorders related to high blood pressure are among the most common medical complications of pregnancy. Because of the unique demands on the circulatory system, women are more likely to develop hypertension during pregnancy than at any other time in their lives. For those whose blood pressure is abnormally high before pregnancy, the problem is likely to become more severe before delivery.

If untreated, hypertension can lead to disorders called pre-eclampsia and eclampsia (described later in this chapter) that endanger both the mother and her unborn baby. More frequently, hypertension interferes with the blood supply to the uterus and, therefore, with the baby's growth. Mild hypertension is not considered dangerous, but the hazards to your baby depend on how high your blood pressure rises and how long it remains elevated. Moderate to severe hypertension causes a significant percentage of fetal growth problems. And as we described in Chapter 8, babies who do not grow well face a much greater risk of complications before, during, and after birth. The womb of a hypertensive mother may become such a hostile environment in the final months of pregnancy that the baby, unable to get the oxygen and nourishment it needs, may die suddenly. There also is a greater risk that the placenta will separate from the uterine wall before delivery (placental abruption).

In the past, the term "toxemia" was used to refer to high blood pressure problems in pregnancy because medical scientists suspected that a toxin, or harmful substance, was at fault. No such culprit has been identified, and the term has been discarded as misleading. But while the terminology has changed, the dangers have not. With early detection and proper treatment, however, you can minimize the risks of high blood pressure. In this chapter we'll review the most common blood pressure abnormalities in pregnancy, the ways in which they're diagnosed, the available treatments, and the prognosis for you and your baby.

· Hypertension in Pregnancy

Pregnancy brings about enormous changes in blood volume and pressure. During the first twenty weeks, blood pressure typically falls below prepregnancy levels. It then begins to rise steadily in the second half of pregnancy, usually back to prepregnancy levels. Blood pressure problems in pregnancy are characterized according to whether they begin before conception or during the first twenty weeks, or after twenty weeks of gestation. "Chronic" hypertension refers to a blood pressure of 150/90 before conception or a reading of 150/90 or an increase of 30/15 over non-pregnant blood pressure after conception and up *to* the first 20 weeks of pregnancy. "Gestational," or pregnancy-induced, hypertension develops *after* the twentieth week of pregnancy or in the first twenty-four hours after delivery. Chronic hypertension is a serious health problem. In most cases, the blood pressure of a woman with gestational hypertension returns to normal shortly after delivery.

Chronic Hypertension

You are more likely to have high blood pressure if you are over 35, smoke, are overweight, have kidney disease, or have a family history of hypertension. Yet you may not find out about your condition until you become pregnant, when the unique physiological demands of carrying a baby may reveal an underlying tendency toward hypertension. Your doctor may become suspicious if your blood pressure reading is high at your first prenatal visit, or if you do not have the typical 10–15 mmHg drop in pressure in the course of early pregnancy. He or she will check your blood pressure frequently. Repeated readings of 150/90 or higher in the first twenty weeks of pregnancy confirm the diagnosis.

If you had high blood pressure before conception or if your blood pressure rises in the first half of your pregnancy, you will have to take precautions to prevent further complications. Ample bed rest and good nutrition are fundamental. Your doctor may advise you to get at least eight hours of rest at night and to spend an extra hour or two lying on either side to enhance blood flow to your baby. Avoid all prolonged vigorous exercise, including strenuous housework and stressful work outside your home. You don't have to restrict your intake of fluids, but you should avoid using more than two grams of salt a day and eat balanced, nutritious meals.

Obstetricians generally use two different types of drugs for chronic hypertension: diuretics, which speed up the elimination of fluids, and antihypertensive medications. Diuretics have a blood pressure–lowering effect of their own; they also maximize the effectiveness of other antihypertensive drugs. However, there is one constraint on their use: When they are begun, they cause a temporary drop in blood plasma and hence in blood volume. This effect lasts for about ten days; then blood volume returns to near normal. The transient decreased blood volume is not considered hazardous to a fetus in the first twenty-four to twenty-six weeks of pregnancy when its total needs are relatively small. But after that point, even a transitory drop in blood volume could interfere with the baby's nourishment and growth. If the baby is already frail and small because of inadequate blood flow to the uterus, the additional stress could jeopardize its survival. To avoid this risk, obstetricians do not usually initiate diuretic treatment after the twenty-fourth to twenty-sixth week. Earlier in the pregnancy, the decision to use diuretics depends on how much and how quickly the mother-to-be's blood pressure is rising.

Antihypertensive drugs do not lower blood plasma or volume, although some of them may interfere with blood flow to the uterus; these are avoided. The most commonly prescribed antihypertension drugs in pregnancy are methyldopa (Aldomet) and hydralazine (Apresoline), which work in a way that does not decrease uterine blood flow. Some physicians prescribe them if diastolic pressure reaches 90 mmHg in the first half of pregnancy; others wait to see if it rises to 110. Obstetricians generally try to stabilize diastolic pressure at about 90, rather than trying to return it to 80 or lower.

Gestational Hypertension

This problem consists of high blood pressure recorded *after* the first twenty weeks of pregnancy or in the first twenty-four hours after delivery. Most women who develop gestational hypertension had normal blood pressures before conception, though some may have an unrecognized predisposition to chronic hypertension. In most cases, blood pressure returns to normal after delivery. You are more likely to develop gestational hypertension if this is your first pregnancy, if you have kidney disease or diabetes, or if you are malnourished. Diagnosis is based on a rise of both systolic and diastolic blood pressure above normal after the twentieth week of pregnancy. One simple screening method is the "rollover' test: You lie on your side on the examining table as your blood pressure is measured. Then you roll onto your back, and another reading is made. Five minutes later—while you're still on your back—your blood pressure is checked again. If the five-minute reading shows an increase of more than 20 mmHg in diastolic pressure, the test is considered positive. As many as 60 to 80 percent of women with positive results develop either gestational hypertension or pre-eclampsia later in pregnancy. But, since 20 to 40 percent of women have falsely positive tests, some doctors do not consider the rollover test useful even as a screening tool.

The basic approach to the treatment of gestational hypertension consists of increased bed rest, good nutrition, and frequent checkups. If your blood pressure is only mildly elevated, you may not be given any medication. Antihypertensive drugs, such as methyldopa and hydralazine, generally are prescribed only if the diastolic blood pressure is over 100.

What to Consider

If your blood pressure rises, the risks to your baby and yourself increase. Excessive pressure on the blood flowing to and through your uterus can interfere with the supply of oxygen and nutrients to your baby because of the associated narrowing of the blood vessels.

Your doctor's primary concerns will be lowering and controlling your blood pressure and preventing pre-eclampsia. If you have hypertension, you should look out for any symptoms that could be early warning signals of pre-eclampsia, including a sudden weight gain, swelling of your fingers or face, headaches, or blurring or dimming of your vision. Call your doctor immediately if any of these symptoms develop.

• Pre-Eclampsia

Pre-eclampsia, an illness unique to pregnancy, consists of hypertension plus edema (retention of fluids) and proteinuria (excretion of protein in the urine because of inadequate kidney function). Like gestational hypertension, pre-eclampsia is both mysterious and distressingly common. It occurs in 5 to 7 percent of all pregnancies of women around the world. This problem is more likely to develop if you are under 18 or over 35 and pregnant for the first time, if you have chronic hypertension, or if you have other complications, such as kidney disease or diabetes.

Pre-eclampsia can range from mild to severe, and the risks to you and your baby also may range from slight to potentially deadly. If you develop the most serious complications of pre-eclampsia, the danger of losing your baby is three times higher than normal. Your own life may be threatened if pre-eclampsia becomes so severe that you experience convulsions; this condition is called eclampsia.

Diagnostic tests for pre-eclampsia include blood pressure measurements, careful recording of weight gain, and analysis of a 24-hour collection of urine. A high urinary protein level indicates poor kidney function. Your blood will be tested for creatinine, a substance normally excreted in the urine; a high blood-creatinine level is another indication that your kidneys are not doing their job.

If you have pre-eclampsia, hospitalization may be necessary to prevent further complications and risks. Initially you will be put on complete bed rest, lying on either side because this may increase blood flow to your uterus and through your kidneys and improve your body's ability to filter wastes. Nutritious meals that are high in protein (70–90 milligrams a day) may help compensate for some of the protein lost in your urine. Women with mild pre-eclampsia who improve after three or four days of this treatment can return home with continuing supervision, including weekly or biweekly tests of blood pressure, weight gain, and kidney function, as well as tests of their babies' well-being. Women with moderate to severe pre-eclampsia have to remain in the hospital for daily evaluation.

If your symptoms are severe and your baby is mature enough to survive outside the womb, an early delivery may be safer for you both. Your obstetrician will weigh the hazards of continued pregnancy against the risks of premature delivery, and may induce labor if the symptoms of pre-eclampsia worsen or the risk of eclampsia increases.

· Eclampsia

Eclampsia is one of the most dangerous complications of pregnancy for both you and your baby. It consists of a combination of severe pre-eclampsia and seizures. There is a 3 to 5 percent mortality rate among women who develop eclampsia and a 20 percent increase in the risk of fetal death. The cause of eclampsia is not known, but the risks seem to be higher in first and twin pregnancies, in women with diabetes, or diseases affecting their blood vessels and in those with a family history of eclampsia.

Eclampsia is a largely—though not entirely—preventable problem, and it is rare in women who are well nourished and receive good prenatal care. Early treatment of chronic hypertension can help minimize the risks. Bed rest and a good diet also may help. If a woman does develop seizures, magnesium sulfate or Valium is used to control them. The only real "cure" for eclampsia is delivery, regardless of the maturity or immaturity of the baby. The risks to the mother's life can be so great that neither she nor the baby would survive if the pregnancy continued. One sign of an urgent need to deliver is a boring pain in the abdomen, which precedes a convulsion. The obstetrician may elect to induce labor if the cervix has begun to soften. If it hasn't, a cesarean delivery may be performed.

· Prognosis

High blood pressure in pregnancy endangers you and your baby. That's why it is so important to take preventive steps, such as making sure you get adequate rest and nutrition. If you can maintain control of your blood pressure throughout pregnancy, you can minimize the hazards.

An unborn baby, totally dependent on its mother for oxygen and nourishment, is particularly vulnerable to problems that impede blood flow. If your blood pressure rises and remains elevated, your baby may not be able to get adequate nutrients and will be small and frail. If hypertension interferes with kidney function in pregnancy, much of the protein your baby needs may be lost in your urine. The dangers to the baby increase as the pregnancy progresses. That is why your doctor will monitor its condition regularly in the last trimester. If survival in the womb becomes too precarious, an early delivery can save your baby's life. Its well-being after birth depends on its maturity and size. The preterm babies of hypertensive mothers seem less susceptible to respiratory problems than other babies born prematurely, but they may require special care for other problems associated with a too-early arrival in the world, such as meconium aspiration or low calcium levels.

Pregnancy does not increase your likelihood of developing hypertension later in life, although it may unmask a predisposition to this problem. Chronic hypertension will persist after delivery and may require continuing treatment. Gestational hypertension usually resolves itself within ten days of delivery, but it may recur in other pregnancies.

Severe pre-eclampsia and eclampsia can endanger your life as well as your baby's. Delivery is the only way of eliminating the risks. Once your baby is born, the symptoms of these disorders ease. None of the hypertensive disorders of pregnancy, including pre-eclampsia and eclampsia, have a lasting impact on blood pressure. Long-term studies document this: there was no evidence of increased hypertension in women who developed eclampsia and were followed for up to forty-four years after delivery. Pre-eclampsia and eclampsia usually do not recur in subsequent pregnancies, unless there is an underlying medical problem or a family predisposition.

12 . Problems of the Heart, Lungs, and Blood

PREGNANCY IS AN EXPERIENCE that quite literally lifts your heart and takes your breath away. Your circulation and respiration change in ways that are as dramatic as the external transformations of your body. During pregnancy your heart enlarges, increasing its output by 30 to 50 percent. As your uterus grows, pushing your diaphragm upward, your heart is lifted and turned slightly. Your chest size and oxygen consumption increase, though you may feel as if you're getting less rather than more air because of the pressure from your growing baby. Your rate of circulation accelerates, and your pulse speeds up by about ten beats a minute. You produce more plasma and blood cells than usual, so your total blood volume increases by more than a third over normal.

As a result of these changes, most pregnant women at times feel breathless or report that their hearts are beating rapidly. At any other time of life, these symptoms might seem ominous. During pregnancy, they are signs of normal physiological adaptation. But if you have an illness that affects your heart, lungs, or blood, the changes and extra demands of pregnancy will require special attention. With precautions and appropriate care, most women with such ailments can have healthy babies and remain healthy themselves. In this chapter we'll describe the most frequent problems affecting the heart, lungs, and blood of pregnant women, their treatments, and their effects on pregnancy.

· Heart Disorders

While changes of the heart are common in pregnancy, heart problems are not. About 1 to 1½ percent of pregnant women have heart disease, usually caused by a congenital defect, rheumatic fever, an abnormality of the heart valves, or an abnormal rhythm.

In the past thirty years, advances in surgery and drug treatment have made repair of many congenital defects possible, so more women born with these problems are surviving into adulthood and becoming pregnant. The possible danger to their unborn babies depends on their hearts' ability to pump an adequate supply of oxygen to the uterus. A very low degree of oxygenation in the mother's blood (a condition called cyanosis) increases the risk of miscarriage and perinatal death. Less severe oxygen deficiencies have been associated with preterm labor and growth impairment.

Rheumatic fever is a delayed result of an infection, usually of the throat, by group A streptococcus bacteria (strep throat). It strikes most often between the ages of 5 and 15 and can be fatal. About half of those who survive develop rheumatic heart disease, a chronic condition caused by scarring and deformity of the heart valves. The incidence of rheumatic fever has declined as antibiotics have been developed that eradicate strep infections before they worsen and spread. The prognosis for pregnancy in a woman with rheumatic heart disease depends on the extent of damage to the heart and, again, on the available oxygen supply for her baby.

The most common disorder of the heart valves in women of child-bearing age involves the mitral valve, which is located on the left side of the heart and keeps blood from going "backward" toward the lung when the heart contracts and pumps blood to the body. If this valve does not close completely, blood will flow backward, making a gurgling sound called a murmur. This is a frequent consequence of rheumatic heart disease, but briefer murmurs also are not uncommon in young women who've never had rheumatic fever. For unknown reasons, a portion of the normal valve is pushed back too far (prolapsed) during the heart's contraction. Particularly if no other symptoms, such as chest pain or a heart rhythm abnormality, occur, mitral valve prolapse is not considered significant before, during, or after pregnancy. Murmurs during the heart's contractions are very common in normal pregnancy, because of the increased flow of blood through the heart, and are of no concern.

Women whose severely diseased or deformed heart valves have been replaced by artificial valves generally require ongoing treatment with drugs called anticoagulants, which prevent blood clots. One widely used agent, warfarin, may cause birth defects if taken in early pregnancy and may increase the risk of hemorrhage if used in the final weeks. Therefore most obstetricians switch to another anticoagulant, heparin, which is considered safe, but must be taken by injection.

The most common heart ailment in our society, coronary artery disease, or atherosclerosis (clogging of the arteries), is rare in pregnant women. Because the chance of developing atherosclerosis increases with age, there is a slightly higher incidence in pregnant women over 35 than in younger mothers.

Evaluating Your Heart's Health

Not even a cardiologist can always know before your pregnancy whether your heart will be able to withstand the stress of childbearing and provide an adequate supply of oxygen to your baby. Your doctor will try to anticipate the potential for any problems by assessing your prepregnancy heart function. Generally, if you have no symptoms or feel chest discomfort only with physical exertion, you should have a relatively uncomplicated pregnancy without any unusual additional risks to you or your baby. The possibility of problems increases if you suffer discomfort or chest pain with less-than-strenuous activity. If you have an extremely incapacitating heart problem, pregnancy can threaten your life as well as your baby's, and a therapeutic abortion and sterilization may be advised if you do become pregnant.

Your obstetrician and cardiologist rely on a variety of diagnostic procedures to learn more about the state of your heart. They can detect some abnormalities by carefully listening to your heart through a stethoscope; however, during pregnancy it becomes more difficult to evaluate heart sounds because the increased amount of blood entering your heart creates a murmur. An electrocardiogram (EKG) records the heart's electrical activity, either at rest or on exertion. In a technique called echocardiography, ultrasound waves produce images of the heart as it pumps. Rarely a potentially ominous problem is evaluated by angiography. In this procedure, a cardiologist threads a tiny tube through the blood vessels to the heart, injects a radiopaque dye, and takes X-rays of the arteries to indicate any blockage or damage.

If you have a heart disorder, a cardiologist will examine you periodically throughout your pregnancy. Close surveillance can detect problems before they worsen and become serious threats to you or your baby.

What to Expect

Even if you have only a mild form of heart disease, your heart may not be able to meet the demands of both pregnancy and physical exertion. To prevent problems, you should restrict your activity. If you have a more serious illness, you may have to spend most or all of your time on bed rest. Try to avoid anxiety and stress, since they can take a toll on your heart. Emotional support from your family and friends may be more important than ever before. Your own commitment and willingness to do what's best for your heart can make a critical difference.

Your obstetrician may advise you to restrict salt intake to two grams a day and to take iron supplements to prevent anemia (page 114). Elastic stockings help prevent pooling of blood in your lower extremities and ease the burden on your heart, particularly in late pregnancy.

You may be given antibiotics as a preventive treatment during any dental surgery, at the first hint of a respiratory or urinary tract infection, and during labor and delivery. Some doctors prescribe antibiotics throughout pregnancy for women with serious valve problems.

If your heart condition is grave, you may be hospitalized for an extended period during your pregnancy to assure continuous care. Very rarely heart surgery, such as replacement of a valve, may be necessary during pregnancy. Such operations pose significant risks of miscarriage, but they have been performed in pregnancies with successful outcomes.

Cardiologists recommend a vaginal delivery, unless obstetrical complications require a cesarean birth. Throughout labor, you'll be given oxygen to alleviate breathlessness, chest pain, and a faster heart rate, as well as medications for pain and anxiety. The obstetrician may use low forceps (see page 180) during delivery to reduce the strain of bearing down and pushing out the baby. The preferred position for delivery is sitting up rather than lying flat. If your legs are elevated for delivery, they will be lowered immediately afterward to reduce drainage of blood into your general circulation. Close monitoring after delivery minimizes the risks of bleeding, infection, shock, or heart failure. If you have moderate to severe heart disease, your doctor may want you to remain in the hospital after the delivery until your heart function returns to normal.

Prognosis

The greatest dangers to the fetus during pregnancy are miscarriage, growth impairment, and preterm birth. If a woman has had one child with a heart malformation, the risk for a subsequent baby can be as high as 5 percent for the more common defects, such as a hole in the wall between the chambers of the heart (the ventricular septum), or only 1 percent for rarer problems. There is no increased risk if the mother or a previous child has had rheumatic heart disease. Your baby's long-term prognosis will depend on its size and maturity at birth.

Within a few weeks of delivery, your heart should return to its normal size, position, and functioning, but the time required for complete recovery depends on the severity of your heart problem. With proper care before, during, and after delivery, you should not sustain any heart damage or long-term impairment. There is no evidence that pregnancy affects life expectancy, except for the most severe heart problems.

· Breathing Problems

The most frequent respiratory problem of pregnancy is dyspnea, the sense of needing to breathe more frequently and deeply. Its cause is unknown, but one suspected culprit is the hormone progesterone. If you have a respiratory illness, breathing difficulties can be more than a temporary discomfort.

Asthma

About 2 percent of all Americans have asthma, and about 0.5 percent of pregnant women are asthmatics. Very often asthma runs in a family, and an inherited disposition to asthma may increase your likelihood of developing wheezing or coughing attacks. Pregnancy's effects on asthma are unpredictable. About a third of asthmatic women get better; a third get worse; a third show no change. Asthma may have no effect at all on pregnancy, particularly if severe attacks are prevented or minimized. Only women with extremely impaired breathing are at higher risk.

If you are asthmatic, you should avoid any possible allergic triggers of attacks and any emotional stresses that may aggravate your condition. You'll be given antibiotics if you develop a respiratory infection. You can use mist and steam inhalers safely throughout pregnancy. The most commonly used asthma medications, including epinephrine, aminophylline, and theophylline, are considered safe in pregnancy. If they are not effective in controlling symptoms, prednisone, a powerful steroid, may be prescribed for a brief period. Its known effects on a human fetus are minimal, but it may reduce birth weight slightly if use is prolonged. Physicians recommend a vaginal delivery. If a cesarean is necessary for obstetrical reasons, you will be given regional rather than general anesthesia to avoid possible respiratory complications.

Pneumonia

Pregnant women are more susceptible to complications from any form of pneumonia—bacterial, viral, or chemical. Because pneumonia can diminish the available oxygen supply, their babies are also at risk. To prevent serious problems, pregnant women are frequently hospitalized for treatment as soon as pneumonia is diagnosed.

Tuberculosis

Fewer than 2 percent of pregnant women in the U.S. have positive reactions to tuberculin skin tests; a much smaller percentage actually develop tuberculosis. TB has no specific effects on pregnancy, and a baby cannot "catch" the disease from its mother before birth. Of the two most commonly used medications to treat TB, rifampin is preferred as safer for use in pregnancy.

· Blood Disorders

Because your production of blood cells increases up to a third above normal during pregnancy, you become more vulnerable to any deficiencies in blood components. The most common of these deficiencies is anemia, caused by low amounts of hemoglobin, the oxygen-carrying component in red blood cells.

Acquired Anemias

Anemia in pregnancy is usually the result of insufficient iron or folic acid. Compared to men, all women have relatively small stores of iron: 200–400 milligrams rather than 1,000 milligrams. During pregnancy, you will need 800 milligrams of iron a day: 300 for your baby and 500 for yourself. This basic requirement is not met in about 20 percent of all pregnancies, resulting in anemia. The growing baby seems to take what it needs from the available iron supply; the mother-to-be is the one who feels the effects of a deficiency. The most common symptom is exhaustion.

Iron-deficiency anemia is diagnosed by a count of your red blood cells. If they make up less than 35 percent of your total blood cells, you are anemic. The usual treatment is a 30- to 60-gram daily iron supplement, which should be taken with foods because it is difficult to digest. Your doctor will determine the amount you take; more iron is not necessarily better. If you cannot tolerate oral doses of iron, injections may be necessary.

Anemia also can be the result of a deficiency of folic acid, an essential nutrient found in leafy green vegetables, kidney and liver meat, and peanuts. Women who do not receive adequate amounts in pregnancy may develop such symptoms as nausea, vomiting, poor appetite, and weight loss. The usual treatment is a daily folic acid supplement. Other acquired anemias, usually associated with inflammatory diseases or reactions to toxic substances, are rare in pregnancy.

Hereditary Anemias

The most common inherited anemia in the U.S. is sickle-cell anemia, a disorder of the hemoglobin in red blood cells that occurs in black Americans and interferes with the normal supply of oxygen to body tissues. In the past, half of the pregnancies of women with sickle-cell disease ended in miscarriage or perinatal death. Today their chances of having a healthy baby are much better.

A major advance in preventing problems for sickle-cell mothers is the use of blood transfusions, beginning in the first trimester and continuing on an average of every one to three weeks. Although some risks are associated with such frequent transfusions, the benefits clearly seem to outweigh them. The perinatal complication and mortality rates of the babies of women who receive regular transfusions during pregnancy has dropped significantly, and growth impairment, once a problem, is prevented.

The main complication for women who have a gene for sickle-cell disease but are not victims of it themselves is infection. If you are a sickle-cell carrier—which can be diagnosed by a blood test at the first prenatal visit—you are almost twice as likely to develop a urinary tract infection before delivery. If not treated promptly and properly, this problem can lead to serious complications for you and your baby (see Chapter 14). Some obstetricians test all sickle-cell carriers for the levels of bacteria in their urine at their first prenatal visit and give preventive antibiotics to those whose high levels indicate a risk of infection.

Beta-thalassemia is another hereditary anemia; it occurs most frequently in families of Mediterranean origin. Women with this problem have small red blood cells and are at higher risk of developing anemia during pregnancy. Iron supplements do not seem to help; transfusions are the standard therapy during pregnancy and delivery.

Other Blood Disorders

Cancers of the blood, such as leukemia and Hodgkin's disease, and clotting disorders, such as thrombocytopenia and polycythemia, are rare conditions among pregnant women. These serious medical problems require individual evaluation and treatment by an obstetrician and a hematologist (a specialist in diseases of the blood).

13 . *Diabetes Mellitus*

ANGELA REGAS was just 10 years old when she found out she had diabetes mellitus. She couldn't understand the long explanations about metabolism and blood sugar levels, but she realized that she was different from other kids. They didn't have to learn how to give themselves shots; they could eat chocolate bars and milk shakes and anything else they wanted. When she heard that diabetics couldn't have babies, she accepted that along with all the other differences that set her apart.

When she was 21, Angela became pregnant. "My initial reaction was panic. I was convinced that the baby would be deformed or that I'd lose my eyesight, so I had an abortion. I didn't think I had any other choice." Now, six years later, Angela wants very much to have a baby. "My doctor told me to forget all those old wives' tales about diabetes and pregnancy. She says I can have a normal baby, but that a lot is going to depend on me."

The chances of successful pregnancy for diabetic women like Angela are indeed better today than ever before. As medical scientists have unraveled the complexities of diabetes mellitus, they have found ways of overcoming many of the risks of pregnancy in diabetics. The perinatal mortality rate in the babies of diabetic mothers has fallen from 30 percent to less than 5 percent in the last three decades. The incidence of birth defects remains higher than in other pregnancies, but a diabetic woman who plans her pregnancy carefully and maintains good control of her metabolism right from the start has an excellent chance of having a normal baby. In this chapter we'll explains what diabetes is, how it affects and is affected by pregnancy, and what you can do to overcome potential risks to your developing baby.

• A Problem of Supply and Demand

Diabetes mellitus affects about 5 percent of all Americans and 1 to 2 percent of pregnant women. Heredity plays some role in the development of diabetes, but its significance is not clearly understood. In mild cases, careful control of the diet may be sufficient to prevent complications. In more serious cases, insulin therapy regulates the metabolism of food. If not treated, diabetes can cause profound changes in many cells and organs of the body, including the eyes, blood vessels, kidneys, and liver.

To understand how diabetes affects the body, you have to understand the basic way in which your body metabolizes, or processes, food. The food you eat is like the gas you put in your car. If this fuel isn't stored and utilized properly, neither your body nor your car can run smoothly. In humans a major fuel for energy production is glucose (sugar). The primary regulator of its storage and metabolism is insulin, a hormone secreted by the pancreas. Normally the level of sugar in your blood rises every time you eat, triggering the release of insulin. By converting the sugar into energy or storing it for future use, insulin brings down the level of sugar in your blood, usually within two hours after eating.

Diabetes interferes with the release of insulin after a meal. In severe cases, the pancreas may produce virtually no insulin at all. Because there isn't enough insulin to metabolize food, the level of sugar in the blood remains high—so high that the kidneys are unable to process all of it and as a result sugar is "spilled" into your urine. A condition similar to starvation develops, no matter how much food you eat, because much of your body's fuel is not being metabolized and used. Deprived of the fuel it needs, your body begins to break down stored fat for energy use; this process produces weak acids called ketones. A buildup of ketones leads to ketoacidosis, an upheaval in the body's chemical balance that brings on nausea, vomiting, abdominal pain, lethargy, and drowsiness. Severe ketoacidosis can lead to coma and eventual death.

Even though diabetes itself is relatively uncommon in pregnancy, changes similar to those associated with diabetes occur in all pregnancies. The developing baby, which also gets much of its fuel from glucose, creates a relative deficiency in your energy supply. If you do not have a steady supply of glucose, you must obtain more and more of your own energy from the breakdown of fats. This increases the risk of ketoacidosis. In the second half of pregnancy, as the demands of your growing baby increase, still more insulin is needed, yet at the same time various hormones produced by the placenta enter your bloodstream and interfere with the action of insulin. Your pancreas is forced to manufacture larger amounts of insulin to meet your and your baby's metabolic requirements.

These added stresses of pregnancy can disturb the basic metabolism to such an extent that they unmask a latent predisposition to diabetes; this problem is described as gestational diabetes. Those women already diagnosed as diabetic before pregnancy frequently have to adjust and readjust their insulin doses, weekly and sometimes daily, to meet the changing needs of their bodies and their babies. The key to successful pregnancy for all diabetics in early evaluation, good control of blood sugar levels, and frequent checkups.

· Gestational Diabetes

The risk of developing diabetes is greater in pregnancy because of the unusual metabolic demands. The risk increases if you have a family history of diabetes; had a baby that was large for its gestational age (over 4,500 grams—10 pounds—at birth); had a previous stillborn or malformed baby or an infant who died within a month of delivery; are overweight, are over 35 years of age; or have an excessive amount of amniotic fluid (hydramnios).

If you meet this risk profile, you'll undergo diagnostic tests early in your pregnancy and again at the twenty-eighth and thirty-second weeks. Some physicians believe that all pregnant women should be screened regularly for abnormal sugar metabolism, especially if they're older than 35.

Diagnosis

There are three standard tests for detecting diabetes in pregnancy: all involve analysis of the levels of sugar in your blood. The simplest and least expensive are a "fasting blood sugar" test, which measures the amount of sugar in your blood before your first meal of the day, and a "postprandial" test, which measures your blood sugar level two hours after a meal. If the results of these tests are inconclusive, your doctor will order a "glucose tolerance test," a series of measurements of blood sugar levels at set intervals after you swallow a prepared sugar solution. This more time-consuming procedure provides definitive information on your metabolism. If your glucose tolerance test is abnormal, you will be diagnosed as having gestational diabetes.

Treatment

Since prevention of further complications is the basic approach to treating gestational diabetes, your blood sugar levels will be checked frequently. Most women who develop gestational diabetes can maintain good control of their metabolism simply by regulating what and when they eat; about 15 percent also require insulin therapy before delivery.

If you develop gestational diabetes, you must pay very close attention to your diet. Rather than eating three big meals, you should have six small ones; this prevents a sudden drop in your blood sugar level. You should try to schedule your meals for approximately the same time every day. Your daily meal plans should consist of 45 to 50 percent carbohydrates, 30 percent fats, and 20 to 25 percent protein.

You usually will be examined at least once very two weeks during your first eight months and weekly thereafter. Your doctor will evaluate your fasting blood sugar levels at every visit. If they are normal, no medical therapy is necessary. If they are too high, you may need insulin therapy. The greatest risk associated with gestational diabetes is not recognizing it. Perinatal mortality is high in diabetic women who do not receive adequate prenatal care and do not have good metabolic control. The risks also increase with the development of other complications, including ketoacidosis (pages 117, 121), pre-eclampsia (Chapter 11), pyelonephritis (Chapter 14), or an excessively large baby.

· Insulin-Dependent Diabetes

If you are diabetic, you should start preparing for pregnancy *before* you conceive. Most physicians recommend that a woman not become pregnant for a year after diabetes is first diagnosed, since the disease is often unstable initially, and blood sugar levels and insulin doses fluctuate. The waiting period also gives you time to become more knowledgeable and confident about coping with diabetes.

Before you attempt to become pregnant, you should establish good metabolic control. Fluctuations in the levels of sugar in your blood increase the risk of congenital malformations and of losing your baby. A blood test that measures hemoglobin A_{lc}, a component of red blood cells, indicates how well you have controlled your blood sugar during the preceding month or two. High levels of this substance very early in pregnancy are associated with an increased likelihood of birth defects. If you consult with your doctor before conception, you can regulate your diet and insulin doses to make sure you are in good metabolic control at the beginning of your baby's life. A hemoglobin A_{lc} test indicating good control is a reassuring way to start a pregnancy.

In general, the outcome of your pregnancy also depends on how long you've had diabetes and whether it has caused any damage to your blood vessels. In order to plan for any possible complications in pregnancy, your physician will classify you according to the severity and duration of your diabetes.

A Matter of Control

The risks to your unborn baby are directly related to your blood sugar levels. As several major research studies have shown, the closer to normal that a diabetic woman's sugar metabolism is kept during pregnancy, the better the outcome. In one report, there was a 4 percent incidence of perinatal death in women whose average blood sugars before eating were kept below 100 mg/dl (milligrams per deciliter, or 100 ccs. of blood); a 16 percent incidence in those with blood sugars of 100–150 mg/dl; and a 24 percent incidence in those with blood sugars above 200 mg/dl.

In order to keep your blood sugars at a low level, you must test your urine and blood frequently. Your renal threshold—the level at which your kidneys begin to spill sugar into your urine—is lower in pregnancy. You should test the amount of sugar and ketones in your urine daily, using the second-voided urine (the urine produced thirty minutes after you first empty your bladder after awakening). Occasionally you may be asked to collect all the urine you produce over a twenty-four period for testing. The standard home urine test for pregnant diabetics is a dipstick method; the most commonly used brand is KETO-DIASTIX. The test involves a chemical reaction between the test tape and a few drops of urine. By comparing the resulting color of the solution to a color chart that comes with the testing kit, you can determine the level of sugar and ketones in your urine.

A more precise way of monitoring your metabolism is to test the amount of sugar in your blood. A new home test method, called a reflectance meter, is simple, easy, and accurate. You prick your finger and smear a drop of blood on a specially prepared test tape. The color change in the strip indicates the amount of sugar in your blood, and the reflectance meter translates the color reaction into a digital readout of your blood sugar level.

The ideal blood sugar level before a meal is 60–100 mg/dl. In order to keep your blood sugar this low, you may have to adjust your insulin doses daily, and keep a careful record of your urine and blood test results. You may need two daily doses of insulin, one before breakfast and one before dinner; occasionally a third injection at noon is necessary. Oral diabetes drugs are not considered safe for your baby and should not be used in pregnancy.

Special Problems

It's not unusual for any pregnant woman to experience some discomforts and risks, but you should be aware of complications that might be more hazardous for you and your baby than they would be for a nondiabetic. For example, morning sickness, a frequent complaint in pregnancy, can create unique problems because it may upset your sugar and insulin needs. You may have to test your sugar levels and adjust your insulin doses much more often than before. Other conditions that you should pay special attention to include:

• *Hypoglycemia.* If your blood sugar levels drop very low, perhaps because of too much insulin, you may become drowsy, nervous, irritable, and weak. You may perspire heavily, feel hungry, and develop a headache or heart palpitations. In severe cases, hypoglycemia can lead to loss of consciousness, coma, or shock because of the lack of available sugar for your brain. Usually you can prevent the more serious symptoms by ingesting a quick supply of sugar, such as fruit juice or a candy bar. In extreme cases, you may require medical treatment.

• *Infection.* Even minor infections of your urinary or respiratory tract can add to the physiological stress on your body and upset insulin requirements. Infections may cause an increased breakdown of fats for energy and increased production of fatty acids and ketones, which can lead to ketoacidosis.

• *Ketoacidosis.* This problem is diagnosed on the basis of high levels of sugar and ketones in your urine and blood. Severe ketoacidosis is considered a medical emergency; during pregnancy, ketoacidosis can become severe and lead to a coma much more rapidly than usual, sometimes in a matter of hours. The risk of ketoacidosis increases after the fifth month; the risk of perinatal death can be as high as 50 percent. The first symptoms are nausea and vomiting, which can cause dehydration. Seek medical care immediately if these symptoms occur.

• *Eye problems.* Diabetes may cause changes in the blood vessels of the eyes that can lead to progressive worsening of your vision. In the past, a woman with early signs of eye damage was considered at higher risk of blindness or vision impairment if she became pregnant. However, if you have proper care and maintain metabolic control, there does not seem to be any increased risk of permanent damage to your eye vessels as a result of pregnancy.

• *Medical complications.* If you have diabetes, the risks to your baby will increase if you develop other problems along the way to delivery. Because diabetes can affect the blood vessels, there is increased risk of gestational hypertension and pre-eclampsia, two disorders related to high blood pressure (see Chapter 11). Hospitalization may be necessary to ensure proper care for you and your baby.

The Risks to Your Baby

The babies of diabetic women often are large for their gestational age. This condition, called macrosomia, makes them more vulnerable, particularly in the last weeks of pregnancy and during delivery. Your doctor can follow your baby's growth by means of serial sonograms (see Chapter 5); this information may be critical if your doctor has to determine if your baby is premature despite its larger-than-normal size.

Diabetic women are at greater risk of having a stillborn baby, and an early delivery may be critical if your baby shows signs of distress in the womb. You should monitor your baby's movements every day; other surveillance tests, including daily measurements of estriol, also may be used (see Chapter 5). If you have very advanced diabetes, testing of your baby's condition may begin as early as your thirtieth week. In more moderate cases, your doctor begins regular monitoring in your thirty-second or thirty-fourth week.

The perinatal mortality rate for babies of diabetic mothers has fallen dramatically in the past decades. The danger of death directly related to blood sugar control is five to ten times higher in the babies of women whose blood sugar levels have been very high throughout pregnancy. About 30 to 40 percent of the babies who die in the perinatal period also have major defects of the heart, central nervous system, skeleton, or kidneys. The risk of birth defects is related to the severity of the mother's diabetes and her metabolic control during early pregnancy.

Because you and your baby may require special care before, during, and after delivery, your doctor may suggest that you transfer to a center with the facilities to provide extra services. Many diabetic women are admitted to the hospital in the last month of pregnancy to ensure closer evaluation of their own and their babies' condition. In the past labor often was induced in the last month; now amniocentesis usually is performed to determine if the baby's lungs are mature. During labor, you may be given a continuous infusion of insulin and glucose to avoid very high blood sugar levels in your body and very low blood sugar levels in your baby. About 50 percent of diabetics have cesarean deliveries, usually because of obstetrical complications or because their babies are so large that they cannot pass through the pelvis safely. A specialist in newborn care frequently is in the delivery room in case the baby needs immediate attention.

· Prognosis

If you develop gestational diabetes, you will be "cured" by delivery. However, the fact that you developed a diabeteslike condition during pregnancy may be a sign of a predisposition to the disease. There is a 20 to 30 percent chance that you will develop overt diabetes eventually, particularly if you are subjected to intense and prolonged physical or emotional stress.

If you were able to control your diabetes by diet alone before pregnancy but needed insulin before delivery, you should be able to return to dietary control once you recover from the metabolic upheaval of having a baby. If you normally use insulin, you'll have to readjust your doses frequently after delivery. Pregnancy will have no long-term effects on your diabetes, unless your blood sugar levels stayed very high. In such instances, there is an increased risk of damage to various organs.

The babies of diabetic mothers are susceptible to a particular array of transitory problems after birth. If delivered early, they may develop respiratory difficulties. About 15 to 50 percent of these babies develop hypoglycemia and have dangerously low blood sugar levels; this deficiency usually is corrected by giving them oral glucose. The babies also are prone to hypocalcemia (low calcium levels) and hyperbilirubinemia (high bilirubin levels that can cause jaundice, which is treated by exposing the baby to light to break down the bilirubin). These problems are generally treated quite easily in an intensive-care nursery, and the prognosis is good. The major long-term threat is that the baby will have a predisposition to diabetes. If the mother alone is diabetic, there is a 20 percent risk; if both parents are, the risk is considerably higher.

14 . Kidney Problems

YOUR KIDNEYS PERFORM a vital function: they remove the waste products of metabolism from your bloodstream and maintain your body's delicate balance of water and salts and acids and bases. During pregnancy, your well-being and your baby's development can depend on how well or how poorly your kidneys do their job.

Each kidney is made up of about a million tubular structures called nephrons. Within each nephron is a ball of capillaries (small blood vessels) called a glomerulus, which filters blood. As the blood passes through the glomerulus, blood cells and large molecules, such as proteins, are retained, while smaller impurities flow into a collecting tubule. This fluid—urine—passes through the ureter into the urinary bladder, where it is stored until you urinate.

A wide range of diseases can affect the kidneys and their ability to process fluids and wastes. Some are acute temporary problems; others are chronic, progressive illnesses that permanently impair kidney function. If you have a kidney disease, you should seek advice about the risks of pregnancy *before* you conceive.

If you have a kidney problem and want to have a baby, your doctor will perform various tests of kidney function, including measurements of the amount of protein "lost" in your urine (proteinuria), the level of creatinine (a substance usually excreted in urine) in your blood, and the rate at which your kidneys process, or clear, wastes from the body (a clearance test).

If your kidneys are only mildly impaired and your blood pressure is normal, you have an excellent chance of having a healthy baby. Pregnancy should not have a long-term effect on your kidneys and will not increase the likelihood of kidney failure. You are more likely to encounter difficulties if your kidney function is poor and if you also have high blood pressure.

Hypertension greatly increases the potential risks of pregnancy for a woman with kidney problems. Many women with severe kidney disease and hypertension (150/190 prior to pregnancy) are unable to conceive. If they do become pregnant, they are at greater danger of developing pre-eclampsia during the second half of pregnancy. This condition can jeopardize a mother's health and her baby's survival in the womb.

Kidney function is so important in pregnancy that if you develop any kidney problems, you should anticipate regular tests for proteinuria, creatinine in your blood, and impaired clearance of wastes. Your doctor also will monitor your blood pressure frequently, because of the double dangers of kidney and blood pressure problems. He or she will try to detect and treat possible complications before they get worse and become more hazardous to you and your unborn baby.

· Urinary Tract Infections

Infections are the most common problems affecting the urinary tract of pregnant and nonpregnant women. Acute infections are caused by bacteria that reach the bladder via the urethra (the tube through which urine passes from the body). As they multiply, bacteria may ascend to the upper urinary tract (the kidneys) and, if not eradicated by antibiotics, may cause chronic problems and increase the risk of preterm labor.

About 5 percent of pregnant women have bacteria in their urine but no symptoms of infection at the time of their first prenatal visit; this condition is detected through routine urinalysis and is called asymptomatic bacteriuria. Approximately 25 percent of this small group of pregnant women will develop symptomatic urine infection before delivery, involving only the bladder or the kidneys as well. However, this risk—and the consequent dangers of preterm labor and perinatal loss—can be overcome by antibiotic therapy. There is only a slight chance of infection in women with no bacteria in their urine at the beginning of pregnancy.

Cystitis

This is the medical term for a bacterial infection of the bladder. While the need to urinate more frequently is normal in pregnancy (because of the pressure of your enlarging uterus on your bladder), you can suspect cystitis if this need becomes even more urgent and particularly if you feel a burning sensation as you urinate. Antibiotics fight the infection, relieve the discomfort, and prevent the spread of the infection to the upper urinary tract.

Pyelonephritis

Acute pyelonephritis is a serious bacterial infection that spreads from the bladder or through the blood vessels and lymphatic system to the kidneys. It occurs in about 2 percent of pregnant women. The symptoms affect the entire body and include fevers, chills, aching pain in the back, loss of appetite, nausea, vomiting, and an abnormally high or low temperature. This problem can be so severe that hospitalization and treatment with high doses of intravenous (IV) antibiotics may be necessary. Most women improve rapidly within two days, but the antibiotics are continued for at least ten days to eradicate all of the bacteria. Repeated urine cultures, or tests, are important after treatment to make sure the acute infection is completely gone, and thus to prevent a chronic infection from developing.

Chronic pyelonephritis is a progressive disease of the kidneys that sometimes occurs after an acute infection, although in other cases its causes are not clear. Since many patients don't notice any early symptoms, doctors often pick up the first indications of this problem during routine testing for proteinuria and hypertension. The impact on your pregnancy depends on how well your kidneys continue to function. If they are clearing wastes and your blood pressure stays normal, your prognosis—and your baby's—is good. Your obstetrician may initiate preventive treatment with antibiotics. A flare-up of this chronic illness is more likely during pregnancy than at other times because of the changes in the body's waste-collecting systems.

· Glomerulonephritis

Glomerulonephritis refers to several different diseases that cause inflammation of the glomeruli in the kidneys. As these ball-like structures are scarred and destroyed, kidney function may deteriorate. The end result can be renal failure, the life-threatening inability of the kidneys to clear wastes and maintain a proper fluid balance.

In chronic glomerulonephritis, fewer and fewer glomeruli are left to filter out waste materials. As a result, there may be high levels of protein in the urine (proteinuria), edema (retention of fluid in body tissues), hypertension, and a buildup of metabolites from amino acid and protein metabolism (azotemia). The outlook for pregnancy depends on whether blood pressure is normal and how much kidney function has been lost. Although doctors have tried many forms of therapy, they haven't found any that is conclusively effective in preventing progression of this disease. Pregnancy does not accelerate the long-term worsening of kidney function. Your obstetrician will weigh the possible benefits of antihypertensive drugs if your blood pressure rises.

Acute glomerulonephritis is an inflammation of the glomeruli of both kidneys. It occurs quite abruptly, often during or after a bacterial infection, such as a strep throat. One clear sign is blood in the urine (hematuria); other symptoms, such as proteinuria and high blood pressure, resemble those of pre-eclampsia, making diagnosis in pregnancy difficult. There is no specific treatment for the inflammation. Hospitalization often is advised for the sake of close monitoring and blood pressure control.

· Nephrosis (Nephrotic Syndrome)

This term refers to a cluster of symptoms of chronic damage to the kidneys, rather than to a particular disease. Very simply, nephrosis consists of chronic proteinuria (the loss of more than one gram of protein a day in the urine), hypercholesteremia (high levels of fats in the blood), and edema (retention of fluid). It may occur in women with chronic glomerulonephritis, systemic lupus erythematosus, diabetes, and syphilis; it also can be a result of poisoning with a heavy metal, such as mercury, some forms of drug therapy, and allergic reactions to insect stings and poison ivy.

If nephrosis occurs prior to a pregnancy, the prognosis largely depends on whether blood pressure is normal. If it is normal, the prognosis is usually good. If, on the other hand, blood pressure is moderately to significantly elevated, the risks increase. If hypertension persists and kidney function deteriorates during pregnancy, the danger of the baby dying in the womb may be so great that immediate delivery is essential, regardless of the baby's gestational age.

Treatment will depend on the underlying cause of nephrosis. Patients who were taking steroids (cortisone) before conceiving may continue this treatment throughout pregnancy. A diet high in protein helps compensate for the protein lost in urine. Your obstetrician will consider the underlying problem that led to nephrosis in determining the best approach for you and your baby.

· Pregnancy After Kidney Failure: Dialysis and Kidney Transplants

The various chronic infectious and inflammatory diseases of the kidney can have the same end result: impairment of the kidneys' ability to process wastes. Occasionally the damage is so severe that the kidneys "fail," or stop working. In rare cases, this can be a consequence of such acute problems as anaphylaxis (an abrupt body-wide allergic reaction to an insect sting or drug), congestive heart failure, or an obstruction. A mechanical process of clearing waste fluids from the body, called dialysis, is used temporarily to do the kidneys' job. Such emergencies rarely occur in pregnancy.

Chronic kidney failure is the result of irreversible damage to the kidneys. In the past, women with severely impaired kidney function did not ovulate or menstruate and therefore did not become pregnant. However, two relatively new treatments for chronic kidney failure—hemodialysis and kidney transplantation—are so effective that women who once were infertile are becoming pregnant. Their risks are undeniably higher than usual, but many of these women are having healthy babies.

Patients on maintenance dialysis rely on machines to filter the waste from their blood by diffusion across a semipermeable membrane. There have been only a few reports of pregnancy in women on maintenance dialysis. In general, the prognosis for pregnancy is not good; nonetheless a number of these women have had successful pregnancies and healthy babies.

An alternative to dialysis for patients with kidney failure is transplantation of a kidney, either from a living, related donor or from a cadaver whose kidney is carefully tissue-matched to the recipient to minimize the risk of rejection. A transplant may be recommended for patients with severely impaired kidney function as a result of infection, chronic inflammation, congenital malformation, trauma, or other diseases that cause irreversible kidney damage.

The prognosis for pregnancy in a woman with a transplanted kidney is brightest if she's been in good general health for at least two years following transplantation, does not have significant hypertension or proteinuria, shows no signs of rejection of the transplant, and is on relatively low doses of the immunosuppressant drugs that prevent rejection. A woman with a transplant from a living relative is less likely to reject the graft and may have a better chance of a successful pregnancy than a woman with a kidney from a cadaver or an unrelated donor. The major risk to the unborn baby is poor growth, particularly if the mother also has hypertension.

· Polycystic Kidneys

In this hereditary disease, normal kidney tissue is gradually encroached upon by multiple cysts of varying size, usually affecting both kidneys. It is rare for the symptoms of this problem—hypertension, proteinuria, and azotemia—to develop before middle age, so this complication is uncommon during the childbearing years. If a pregnant woman should develop the signs of this disease, the outlook for pregnancy depends on the extent of hypertension and kidney impairment.

· Kidney Stones

The formation of "stones" within the kidneys does not happen often in pregnancy, but women who've had kidney stones before are likely to develop them again, whether they're pregnant or not. Usually the stones do not obstruct the flow of urine or interfere with kidney function, but infection can develop behind a stone. Ultrasound can detect many stones, but occasionally a doctor will order X-rays to confirm or rule out a problem. Any obstructions that do occur tend to be temporary, and the stones are eventually passed in the urine. If necessary, they may be removed surgically or through a tube inserted through the bladder. There is increased risk of preterm labor during an acute attack, but the usual medical approach is a conservative one of waiting for the stones to pass spontaneously. Pain medications are frequently necessary.

15 . Illness and Pregnancy

NOT VERY LONG AGO pregnancy seemed to be an extremely hazardous venture for many women with chronic diseases. Often these women felt they would have to make a cruel choice between having a healthy child and staying healthy themselves. But because of advances in medical understanding and therapy, women who might once not have dared to conceive are becoming pregnant—and with proper care, giving birth to healthy babies.

In this chapter we will describe some of the more prevalent chronic illnesses of women in their childbearing years, and we'll also discuss some temporary problems that can complicate a pregnancy.

· Thyroid Problems

Pregnancy induces major changes in the thyroid gland and the hormones it produces. In a small percentage of women, the thyroid hormones become abnormally high, resulting in a condition called hyperthyroidism (too much thyroid hormone). It may be difficult to diagnose this problem in pregnancy because the symptoms are similar to such normal changes as a feeling of excessive warmth, nervousness, and a rapid pulse. The most striking signs are a fast heart rate (tachycardia) and a failure to gain weight despite a good appetite. Your doctor will measure the levels of the various thyroid hormones in your blood to arrive at the diagnosis.

Because hyperthyroidism is a danger to the mother's and the baby's well-being, treatment is essential. Some standard medications, such as iodides and propranolol, are not used because they can cause birth defects. The most widely used drugs for controlling hyperthyroidism in pregnancy are propylthiouracil and methimazole (Tapazole); they inhibit the synthesis of thyroid hormones. Your doctor will monitor the dosage carefully and usually will taper it in the final weeks to lessen the risks of complications from abnormal thyroid function in the baby after birth. If the hyperthyroidism is severe ("thyroid storm"), it may be necessary to administer iodides, which block the release of thyroid hormone. However, the iodides can cause a thyroid goiter (enlargement of the gland) and hypothyroidism in the fetus, so they must be used with caution and only when absolutely essential. If medical treatment is not effective, surgical removal of thyroid gland is occasionally necessary. The optimum time for such surgery is the midtrimester, because of the danger of miscarriage in the first trimester and of preterm labor in the third. After this operation, oral doses of thyroid hormone maintain the normal levels essential for the mother's proper functioning. All newborns of mothers with hyperthyroidism must be watched very carefully for neonatal hypothyroidism in the first days after delivery. In follow-up studies, babies born to women treated for hyperthyroidism while pregnant have not shown any physical or intellectual abnormalities in their development, if any thyroid disorders they develop are treated promptly.

Pregnancy is relatively uncommon in women with very low thyroid hormone levels (hypothyroidism), because infertility frequently is associated with this disorder. If a hypothyroid woman does become pregnant, she continues thyroid-replacement therapy. This hormone does not cross the placenta and poses no danger to the growing baby. There is a slightly increased risk of miscarriage or perinatal loss, but no reported increases in defects or abnormal development of the babies.

· Digestive Problems

Heartburn, indigestion, nausea, and vomiting are frequent complaints in pregnancy because of normal changes in the digestive tract. As the uterus grows, it presses against your stomach, sometimes forcing stomach acid up into your esophagus and causing a burning sensation. Nausea and vomiting occur in about 40 percent of pregnancies in the first trimester—and not just in the morning. Usually you can cope with these problems by changing your eating habits as described in Chapter 3. For severe nausea and vomiting, the most widely used treatment is a combination of vitamin B_6 and an antihistamine, or vitamin B_6 alone.

There are a number of more serious and unusual complications of the digestive tract which require attention in pregnant women.

Hyperemesis Gravidarum

This ailment is characterized by extremely severe nausea and vomiting, usually in the first trimester although it can occur at any time in a pregnancy. As a result of persistent vomiting, the mother-to-be may lose weight and become dehydrated, disrupting the body's balance of fluids, electrolytes, and acids. Hospitalization and administration of intravenous fluids may be necessary to restore normal metabolic balance and prevent serious liver damage. Psychological factors play an important role in this disorder, particularly when the pregnancy is unwanted or illegitimate. Counseling may decrease the severity of the symptoms and help the woman sort out her feelings about becoming a mother.

Appendicitis

Appendicitis occurs once in every 2,000 pregnancies; the greatest danger is failing to recognize and treat it. In pregnancy, diagnosing appendicitis can be difficult because the symptoms—loss of appetite, nausea, vomiting, abdominal discomfort—are common complaints of mothers-to-be. The typical pain and tenderness are not felt in the usual site but higher up, because the appendix is pushed upward and farther toward the back as the uterus grows. The longer the delay in making the diagnosis and removing the appendix, the greater is the risk of complications. There is increased risk of preterm labor with an appendectomy, as with any abdominal surgery, particularly in the last trimester, but the risks of a ruptured appendix to mother and baby are far graver.

Inflammatory Bowel Disease

Ulcerative colitis and Crohn's disease, both inflammations of the bowel, are not uncommon problems for women of childbearing age. Both diseases usually begin before age 40; the typical sign is chronic diarrhea, which may be bloody in colitis patients. In Crohn's disease, abdominal pain, fever, loss of appetite, and weight loss may occur along with diarrhea. In most people, inflammatory bowel disease remains a lifelong problem, with occasional flare-ups and, particularly in ulcerative colitis, progressive worsening.

The course of these diseases seems to be independent of pregnancy. Pregnancy does not appear to affect them, and they do not affect the outcome of pregnancy if well controlled. Usually a woman with either problem continues to take the same medications she did before conception. The most commonly used agents are corticosteroids. If they are used, the baby may be slightly smaller than usual. Without prompt treatment, an acute flare-up of either condition can jeopardize the unborn baby and increase the danger of infection and preterm labor. If a woman has active symptoms throughout pregnancy, she may become worse after delivery.

Gallbladder Disease

The gallbladder is a sac attached to the underside of the liver that stores bile, a bitter, greenish-yellow liquid secreted by the liver, and aids in digestion of fats. Occasionally cholesterol forms small stones within the gallbladder that can block the flow of bile from it. An estimated fifteen million Americans have gallstones, and women are twice as likely as men to develop them. Their incidence in pregnancy is not known, since they often are not detected. There is no evidence that pregnancy actually causes gallstones, but the gallbladder does become sluggish as a result of the normal physiological changes of pregnancy. If bile is not completely emptied from it, there is greater risk of gallstone formation. The characteristic symptom of gallstones is chronic pain in the upper right side of the abdomen, with attacks lasting fifteen to sixty minutes and recurring episodically. Ultrasound can detect 97 percent of all gallstones, and X-rays are rarely needed.

If you develop gallstones in pregnancy, you will receive the same treatment you would at any other time: drugs for pain relief. Your obstetrician also may observe you closely for signs of preterm labor. About a quarter of the women who already have gallstones become worse in pregnancy. Most doctors take a conservative approach to an attack, advising hospitalization, intravenous medications, and emptying the stomach by means of a suction pump. If surgery is necessary to remove the stones, the risks of miscarriage or preterm labor are lowest in the midtrimester.

Another potential problem is cholecystitis, an inflammation of the gallbladder that can be either acute or chronic. An acute attack usually is caused by a gallstone obstructing the outlet of the gallbladder; symptoms include nausea, vomiting, and flatulence. Chronic cholecystitis typically develops slowly, usually in people who also have gallstones, and causes pain that may be mild to excruciating. In severe cases, surgical removal of the gallbladder may be advised.

Pancreatitis

Inflammation of the pancreas is a rare but serious complication that is more likely to occur in pregnant women with gallstones, infections, or pre-eclampsia, or in pregnant alcoholics. The primary danger is that diagnosis will not be made quickly, and it is compounded by the fact that diagnosis is difficult in pregnancy because the symptoms—nausea, vomiting, abdominal pain, and fever—often occur in normal pregnancies. Treatment consists of "putting the pancreas to rest" for several days by witholding foods and providing intravenous fluids and hospital care. Unrecognized and untreated pancreatitis can cause hemorrhaging (excessive bleeding) of the upper digestive tract and shock, grave dangers to both mother and child.

· Liver Problems

Hepatitis

This viral infection of the liver has two forms: hepatitis A, transmitted by fecal contamination of food or water, and hepatitis B, transmitted by body secretions of fluids, such as blood, semen, saliva, and breast milk.

Hepatitis can incubate for two to six months; a carrier of the disease who never develops symptoms may transmit it to others. The early signs are nausea, vomiting, chills, fever, and diarrhea. The liver becomes enlarged and tender; sometimes the yellowish tinge of jaundice appears. Most pregnant women with hepatitis are hospitalized for supportive care, primarily bed rest and a high-protein diet. If vomiting persists, intravenous fluids may be given. A pregnant woman living in the same house as a person with active hepatitis should ask her doctor about a preventive injection of gamma globulin.

Prompt treatment of hepatitis lowers the risks of perinatal death, preterm delivery, and growth impairment. Occasionally babies acquire hepatitis in the womb; they also are susceptible after birth and may be isolated from their mothers and given gamma globulin to prevent serious complications. Some infants do not develop any symptoms but become carriers of the disease.

Cholestasis of Pregnancy (Icterus Gravidarum)

This problem, sometimes referred to as pregnancy jaundice, consists of itching and/or jaundice caused by pregnancy-induced changes that impair or block the flow of bile in the liver. As the levels of two components of bile—bilirubin and bile salts—increase, the skin may turn yellow, which is characteristic of jaundice, and itch intensely. This usually begins in the third trimester. The liver itself does not become inflamed and is not damaged.

There is no specific treatment for this disorder, and the symptoms disappear after delivery. If the itching becomes unbearable, the obstetrician may prescribe cation exchange resins (cholestyramine) to relieve the irritation. Side-effects are minimal. Several studies of pregnant women with this ailment, particularly those with jaundice as well as itching, have found a higher incidence of fetal growth impairment, preterm labor, and perinatal death, as well as of maternal hemorrhage after delivery. However, researchers do not know exactly how changes within the liver may increase the risks to the unborn baby or the mother.

A woman who develops jaundice and itching in one pregnancy is likely to have the same problem in subsequent pregnancies. Similar symptoms have occurred in women taking oral contraceptives containing high doses of estrogen.

· Autoimmune Disorders

The immune system is a complex and elegant defensive network that protects the body from a host of dangers. At times, however, it fails to recognize the tissues of the body as "self" and attacks them as if they were invading threats. The resulting problems are called autoimmune disorders. Many of these diseases strike otherwise healthy women, most often in their reproductive years.

Systemic Lupus Erythematosus (SLE)

"SLE," or lupus, is an inflammatory disorder of the connective tissue that occurs predominantly in young women; 90 percent of its victims are females. It may begin abruptly with a fever and be mistaken for an infection. Sometimes the disease progresses insidiously for months or years with episodes of fever and malaise as the only symptoms. Eventually most patients experience arthralgia, or pain in their joints and connective tissue; some develop a characteristic butterfly-shaped red rash on their faces, along with other skin changes that intensify in sunlight. SLE can produce damage in various organ systems, including the heart, blood vessels, and kidneys. Diagnosis is based on clinical symptoms, evidence of kidney disease and blood changes, and identification of a lupus "factor," an autoantibody associated with SLE, in the blood. The typical course of this chronic disease includes periodic flare-ups and remissions.

About 1 of every 400 women of childbearing age has SLE. Its impact on pregnancy is unpredictable. About a third of affected women improve; a third show no change; a third get worse, particularly in the first and third trimesters. Severe flare-ups are most likely after delivery. About 10 to 30 percent of all cases of SLE begin during or just after pregnancy.

In general the effects of SLE on pregnancy are more worrisome than the effects of pregnancy on SLE. The miscarriage rate is high: 20 to 30 percent. There also is a somewhat higher risk of stillbirths. About a third of the babies of women with SLE are born prematurely, and the newborns also tend to be small for their gestational age.

The chance for a successful pregnancy is considerably better if SLE is in remission at the time of conception, and if the woman has no evidence of high blood pressure or kidney disease. The treatment of SLE is always individualized according to the severity of the symptoms and the patient's condition. In order to prevent flare-ups, most patients receive ongoing treatment with immunosuppressant (cortisone-like medications) drugs, which inhibit the normal responses of the immune system. Their continued use in pregnancy is controversial, because balancing the potential risks and benefits is difficult and often not clear. Prednisone, a corticosteroid, is the most commonly used immunosuppressant. Babies of women who take prednisone during pregnancy are slightly smaller than normal. A flare-up of SLE poses a much greater danger to their survival than does this growth impairment.

Some obstetricians administer additional corticosteroids during labor to prevent adrenal insufficiency during the period of stress and flare-up after delivery. Because of the risks to the unborn baby in the final weeks of pregnancy, your doctor may advise frequent testing of its well-being and, if necessary, an early delivery.

The lupus factor has been found in babies' umbilical cords and blood after birth, suggesting transmission across the placenta from mother to fetus. However, newborns rarely, if ever, exhibit any clinical signs of the disease.

Rheumatoid Arthritis

In this autoimmune disorder, the body attacks its own connective tissue, causing soreness and damage in the joints. Rheumatoid arthritis is the most common form of arthritis and affects 1 percent of the population, striking women two or three times more often than men. It may develop at any age, but usually is diagnosed between the ages of 35 and 45. Osteoarthritis generally strikes later in life and is rare in pregnancy.

The primary symptoms are pain and tenderness, sometimes only in certain joints, such as those of the hand, and sometimes in all of the most active joints, including the feet, wrists, elbows, and ankles. In some cases, diagnosis is based on identification of rheumatoid factors, or antibodies, in the blood. In other patients, the characteristic symptoms confirm the diagnosis, whether or not there are antibodies in the blood.

The severity of the symptoms determines the need for therapy, and there is a wide range of treatments. The most frequently used drugs are the salicylates, such as aspirin, for relief of inflammation. Occasionally arthritis improves dramatically during pregnancy, with the same easing of pain and soreness that occurs in a spontaneous remission. About a third of pregnant women report no change, and a third become worse. There does not seem to be any increased risk to the baby because of arthritis and its treatment. However, high doses of aspirin or other salicylates in the last trimester increase the risk of prolonged gestation and of maternal and newborn hemorrhage at delivery.

Myasthenia Gravis

In this uncommon autoimmune disorder, the body attacks cells involved in muscle function, causing various degrees of muscle weakness. Myasthenia may begin suddenly or progress slowly for some time. The first muscles affected usually are those of the eyelids and face; gradually fatigue and weakness worsen. Myasthenia is a problem in pregnancy only in its severe forms.

Pregnancy's effects on myasthenia are variable. Flare-ups seem more likely in the first trimester and after delivery. At delivery the obstetrician is extremely cautious about the use of anesthesia, because it may have a prolonged and profound effect on maternal breathing.

A mother may transfer her antibodies against muscle and nerve cells to her unborn baby. About 10 to 20 percent of infants of mothers with myasthenia show temporary symptoms, including weak muscles in the face and limbs, difficulty in swallowing, and weak crying and sucking. They may be admitted to the intensive-care nursery for close observation. Usually the symptoms disappear in four to six weeks.

Disorders of the Reproductive Organs

Endometriosis is a relatively common problem in which cells from the endometrium, the lining of the uterus, migrate to other locations within the pelvis. It occurs most often between the ages of 30 and 40; its causes are not known. Endometriosis is more of a threat to fertility than to successful pregnancy, though in women who do conceive there is increased risk of ectopic pregnancy (see Chapter 7). In most women, endometriosis improves during pregnancy. *NO.*

Fibroid tumors, or myomas, are benign growths of muscle within the uterus. If you have fibroids, the risk of infertility, miscarriage, and preterm labor will depend on their number, size, and location in your uterus. Occasionally fibroids become larger during pregnancy, causing severe pain as they outgrow their available blood supply. In such cases, hospitalization and pain therapy may be necessary. Very rarely a fibroid blocks the baby's passage from the uterus, and a cesarean delivery is necessary. If you have multiple large fibroids or a history of repeated miscarriages or preterm labor, you can undergo a myomectomy, surgical removal of the growths, *before* you become pregnant.

An estimated 1 in every 300 women has a uterine anomaly, or malformation. The uterus may be divided into two compartments (a septate uterus), or it may be forked (bicornuate), or there may be two complete or partial reproductive tracts. If the defect is relatively minor, the prognosis for a successful pregnancy is excellent. Overall, however, there is a higher risk of miscarriage, growth impairment, and preterm labor in women with such problems.

Ovarian cysts often impair fertility. In women who do conceive, they generally have no effect on a pregnancy, although large cysts may make it difficult for the obstetrician to check on the size of the uterus and the baby's growth. Depending on their size and location, cysts may interfere with normal progress during labor, and a cesarean delivery may be necessary. The obstetrician may advise surgical removal of a very large cyst because it might be malignant.

Exposure to DES (diethylstilbestrol) in utero can cause anatomical changes in the reproductive tract. Several studies have also linked prenatal DES exposure to problems of infertility, miscarriage, and preterm labor in DES daughters because of the DES-induced alterations. However, the majority of DES daughters eventually do become pregnant and have healthy babies. The chance for successful pregnancy depends on the particular effects the DES has had on the reproductive organs. Occasionally the cervix is incompetent (unable to hold the growing fetus and amniotic sac). A suture placed around the cervix can strengthen it (see Chapter 7).

· Skin Problems

Changes in your skin during pregnancy, particularly increased pigmentation, are normal. The skin around the nipples of your breasts darkens, and the "linea nigra," or dark line, becomes visible from the top of your abdomen to your pubic bone. In some women, brownish splotches appear on their cheeks, forming the so-called mask of pregnancy. As the skin of your abdomen expands, fine silvery lines may appear; unlike the other pigmentation changes, these stretch marks usually do not disappear after delivery.

More serious and troublesome skin problems also may appear in pregnancy, including intense itching that can extend over the entire body or be localized in the genital region. In a few women, the itching becomes so intense that they cannot sleep or rest. At least in some cases, estrogen-induced increases in the level of bile salts produced by the liver are responsible for the itching. Little can be done to relieve it, although some topical medications can be soothing; your obstetrician can suggest what is best for you. Your doctor may prescribe cation exchange resins if the itching is due to icterus gravidarum (page 134).

Occasionally itchy blisters or minute plaques and papules appear in pregnancy, spreading over the abdomen, thighs, buttocks, arms, and legs. The itching and blisters disappear soon after delivery, but they may recur in a subsequent pregnancy. Usually the baby is not affected.

Venereal warts (condylomas) are highly infectious sexually transmitted growths that appear on the labia. For unknown reasons, pregnancy seems to stimulate their growth. The usual treatment in nonpregnant women is a drug called podophyllin, but it is not used in pregnancy because of its potential hazards to the fetus. Topical preparations can provide some relief, but you should consult your doctor before using them.

The skin problems associated with herpes simplex, an infection which also causes lesions on the genitals, are discussed on page 148.

• Neurological Disorders

Epilepsy

One-half to 1 percent of all Americans suffer from disorders of brain function that cause recurring, sudden attacks of violent muscle contractions and/or unconsciousness. Epilepsy, derived from the Greek word for seizure, is the term used to refer to a variety of seizure disorders.

Seizures generally are characterized as major, or grand mal; minor, or petit mal; and psychomotor. A grand mal seizure is generalized; that is, it affects the entire body. The person loses consciousness, falls to the ground, and experiences convulsive body movements. The seizure may begin with a sinking or rising sensation, called the aura, and may last for two to five minutes. Petit mal seizures are briefer, characterized by a loss of consciousness for ten to thirty seconds, eye or muscle flutterings, and occasionally a loss of muscle tone. They occur predominantly in children. A psychomotor seizure involves both mental processes and muscular movements, such as confusion accompanying a physical activity. For a period of one or two minutes, the individual may stagger, utter unintelligible sounds, and perform automatic, purposeless movements. He or she cannot understand what is said and may resist aid. About 90 percent of epileptics experience grand mal seizures, either alone or in combination with other types. Diagnosis is based on a history of recurring attacks and a study of the brain's electrical activity, called electroencephalography (EEG).

About half of cases of epilepsy are of unknown origin; they are classified as idiopathic epilepsy. All others are symptomatic of conditions that affect the brain, such as trauma, tumors, congenital malformations, or inflammation of the membranes covering the brain. Idiopathic epilepsy usually begins between ages 2 and 14. Seizures before age 2 are usually related to developmental defects, birth injuries, or a metabolic disease affecting the brain. (Fever-induced convulsions bear no relationship to epilepsy.) After age 14, seizures generally are symptoms of a brain disease or injury. Seizure disorders do not reflect or affect intellectual or psychological soundness, and persons who suffer from them are of normal intelligence.

Therapy with anticonvulsant drugs is remarkably effective in controlling seizures. Since no single drug controls all types of seizures, the choice of drug is individually determined; and some patients require several daily drugs. Once seizures are under control, epileptics can live full, normal lives.

An estimated 1 of every 200 pregnant women has a seizure disorder. The major concern for them, and their obstetricians and neurologists, is controlling the seizures without creating risks for the unborn baby. Like other drugs that are beneficial to adults, some anticonvulsants can have adverse effects on fetal development. The most commonly prescribed anticonvulsants are the hydantoins; the best-recognized trade name among this family of drugs is Dilantin. Ninety to 95% of Dilantin users bear completely normal babies. However, other hydantoins can cause fetal hydantoin syndrome, a cluster of birth defects that includes growth impairment, mental deficiency, and facial malformations. Some affected babies also have cleft lips and palates and heart defects. Another anticonvulsant, Tridione (trimethadione), can cause similar defects. As many as 80 percent of the babies of mothers who take this drug have impaired physical and intellectual development, unusual facial features, cleft palates, and heart defects.

If you have been taking these anticonvulsants, your doctor may recommend either that you stop use of any anticonvulsant or that you switch to another drug. Some pregnant women remain free of seizures without any medication; most do require treatment for seizure control. You, your obstetrician, and your neurologist will have to work out carefully the approach that is best for you and your baby. It is critical that your seizures be prevented or controlled because they temporarily interfere with the oxygen supply to the uterus and fetus, thereby endangering your baby.

The drug currently considered safest in pregnancy is phenobarbitol, a barbiturate. While there is some concern that this drug may interfere with growth, the danger seems to occur only with very high doses. If you are given phenobarbitol, you will undergo frequent blood tests to monitor the amount of the drug in your body, and doses will be carefully regulated. With careful control of seizures, epileptic women do not have a higher rate of complications or miscarriages, malformations, premature labor, or perinatal death.

Headaches and Migraines

Headaches are common complaints in pregnancy; usually they are not serious. However, a sudden, intense headache in the second half of pregnancy may be a warning signal of pre-eclampsia, a problem related to high blood pressure (see Chapter 11).

Talk to your doctor before you take *any* pain-relieving medications for headache. Aspirin, the most popular headache remedy, can cause prolonged gestation and increased bleeding at delivery if taken in high doses in the last trimester. Your doctor may recommend an alternate drug.

Migraine headaches are characterized by severe pain on one side of the head and may be accompanied by nausea. The standard treatment in nonpregnant women often involves drugs containing ergotamine, a caffeinelike substance that causes contractions of the uterus. You should *not* use such medication during pregnancy because of the risk of preterm labor; ask your obstetrician for substitute remedies.

Other Neurologic Problems

Women whose lower limbs are paralyzed, whether as a result of an accident or polio, generally can conceive and bear healthy children. They are at greater risk of urinary tract infections and problems caused by continuous pressure on their skin. Labor may be painless but prolonged, because they may not be able to help push the baby through the birth canal.

Multiple sclerosis is a slowly progressive disease of the central nervous system that causes demyelination (destruction of the sheath that covers nerve fibers) of the spinal cord and brain, resulting in symptoms that range from weakness or clumsiness in a hand or leg to loss of sensation and movement. The course of the disease is unpredictable. Some patients have a single episode; others have frequent attacks. Only 1 in every 4,000 pregnant women has multiple sclerosis, and usually the outlook for mother and baby is good.

16 . Infection and Pregnancy

JERRY JOHNSTON is a pleasant young man with reddish brown hair and gray eyes. Most other 17-year-olds, perched at the verge of adulthood, are preoccupied with cars, girls, and sports. Jerry doesn't drive, has never had a date, and doesn't play softball, or basketball. Unlike other adolescents, his future is not filled with the promise of seemingly endless tomorrows. His world exists only in the present.

Six months before his birth, Jerry's mother contracted rubella (German measles). Her symptoms were so mild that she dismissed them as the signs of a cold, but the impact of the virus on her unborn baby was devastating. He was born deaf, blinded by cataracts, and mentally retarded.

Jerry was among 30,000 infants born with deformities following a nationwide rubella epidemic in 1964–65. A tragedy for many thousands of American families, that outbreak also marked the beginning of the end of the threat of rubella. For the first time scientists were able to see the direct relationship between the virus and birth defects. Applying their new understanding of the disease, they devised tests to identify mothers at risk and, in 1969, developed a vaccine to protect them.

Rubella is only one of the infectious diseases that can threaten unborn children, particularly in the first three months of pregnancy. During this time of rapid growth, damage to just a few cells as a result of infection can mean the loss or impairment of an entire line of cells. In this chapter we'll describe the viral, bacterial, and other infections that can endanger an unborn baby.

· Rubella (German Measles)

If you are exposed to rubella virus—whether or not the flulike symptoms (headache, fever, swollen glands, malaise, and rash) are apparent—you develop antibodies that will protect you permanently against another bout with the virus. A simple blood test, in some states required by law of all women applying for a marriage license, detects such antibodies and indicates whether you, and any children you may conceive, are susceptible. If you are, rubella vaccine, which contains a live but greatly weakened strain of the virus, stimulates the development of antibodies to protect you against future infection.

Since massive rubella vaccination began in 1969, some 80 percent of children between the ages of 5 and 9 and 66 percent of those between 1 and 4 have been immunized. The goal is vaccination of every girl before adolescence. Despite this campaign, the Centers for Disease Control estimate that 15 to 20 percent of women of childbearing age are at risk—a higher percentage and total number than the 10 percent of women who were vulnerable in 1964. Because there have not been any national epidemics since then, fewer persons have been exposed to the disease and have thereby developed antibodies. Many would-be mothers who were teenagers in the 1960s have been neither vaccinated nor exposed.

If a woman with no rubella antibodies contracts the virus during pregnancy, there is a 10 to 15 percent chance that her baby will be born with deformities. The risks are not related to the severity of the disease in the mother, but to the timing of exposure to the virus. During the first trimester, half of the babies whose mothers contract rubella may be born with severe effects of heart, eyes, and brain. The incidence and severity of problems are lower if the infection strikes in the second and third trimesters, but they still exist.

About 30 percent of babies exposed to the rubella virus before birth die in the first four months of life. Some of the survivors may require institutional care all their lives. Others suffer lingering effects that are not recognized for months or years. Heart disorders may not be detected immediately. Hearing loss often isn't noticed until the baby is a year or two old. Mild mental retardation and learning disabilities frequently are not diagnosed until the child enters first grade.

You will be checked for rubella antibodies in your blood at your first prenatal visit. Vaccination in the first three months of pregnancy is at least theoretically hazardous, because the fetus would be exposed to a form of the virus; in fact, however, there have been no reports of damage in children whose mothers were vaccinated in error shortly before or early in pregnancy. If a woman is exposed to rubella and is uncertain whether or not she is vulnerable, a sensitive test can determine whether she is immune. A susceptible woman who develops rubella in the first trimester may choose to have a therapeutic abortion.

· Cytomegalovirus (CMV)

This virus, which can cause as much damage as rubella, if not more, is the most common prenatal infection today, though many people have never heard of it. Antibodies to cytomegalovirus are detected in the blood or urine of 3 to 5 percent of pregnant women; an estimated 5,000 to 8,000 babies are affected by this disease each year. If a woman who has had a CMV infection has a recurrence during pregnancy, the risk of infection in her baby is much less than it is if a woman has her first CMV infection during pregnancy.

In adults cytomegalovirus may produce symptoms that mimic mononucleosis, or it may be totally asymptomatic. In an unborn child, the effects include brain damage, retardation, liver disease, cerebral palsy, auditory defects, cardiac defects, and other developmental abnormalities. The consequences of infection may be as dangerous in the second trimester as in the first.

There is no treatment or vaccine for cytomegalovirus, so the only hope is prevention. Researchers know that adults can transmit the infection by virus shed from the nose or mouth or by sexual contact. The infection is more common in crowded and unsanitary living conditions, and good hygiene and sanitation are recommended preventive steps.

Approximately 0.5 to 1 percent of newborns secrete cytomegalovirus from the mouth, nose, or urine at birth. However, only 10 percent of these babies ever develop the severe neurological signs of the disease. Babies infected in the third trimester or during birth (because the virus is on the mother's cervix) may show no detectable signs for several years, when problems such as impaired hearing, diminished intelligence, and weakened immunity become apparent. The prognosis for a child exposed to cytomegalovirus before birth is good if neurological development at age 2 is normal.

· Other Viral Infections

During pregnancy you are more susceptible to viral infections, including the common cold and flu, and more likely to develop complications once infected. If you don't get prompt treatment, a minor cold will sometimes turn into a severe respiratory infection. If you take good care of yourself, there should be no effect on your growing baby. Don't take any over-the-counter cold or cough remedies without your doctor's approval. You also should avoid preventive shots, such as flu vaccinations, unless you have a chronic respiratory condition and your doctor recommends them.

Since most adult women have had measles and mumps as children, they are unlikely to come down with these problems in pregnancy.

There is greater concern about another common childhood hazard, chickenpox. It is not considered harmful through most of pregnancy, but if a woman is infected with chickenpox (varicella) virus within four days of delivery, her body will not have time to manufacture protective antibodies and pass them on to her baby. That means the newborn baby may catch chickenpox at birth and not have any natural immunity against it. If this happens, your baby may be given protective gamma globulin to decrease the risk of infection.

• Bacterial Infections

The most common bacterial infections in pregnancy occur in the urinary and the lower reproductive tracts. They can be hazardous to an unborn baby if they aren't recognized and treated properly.

It is not at all unusual for bacteria to be found in your vagina—whether or not you're pregnant. Most of these microbes pose no danger to you or your baby. However, if one particular type of bacteria, group B streptococcus, is the predominant microorganism in your vagina, the risk of neonatal infection increases. Group B strep is one of the most lethal threats to newborns. Antibiotics given to a mother with a positive vaginal culture may decrease the likelihood of neonatal infection.

The risk of infection increases if the amniotic membranes rupture more than twenty-four to seventy-two hours prior to the beginning of labor. Some physicians try to prevent a neonatal bacterial infection by administering antibiotics if the mother's membranes do rupture prematurely, but there is little evidence that this is effective.

It is much less common to find bacteria in the urine of pregnant women than in their vaginas. At their first prenatal visits, only 5 percent of mothers-to-be have bacteria in their urine; about 25 percent of those eventually develop a symptomatic infection. To prevent this risk—and the subsequent dangers of preterm labor and perinatal loss—antibiotics may be given to eradicate the bacteria. Urinary tract infections are unlikely in women who have no bacteriuria early in pregnancy. The various bacterial infections of the urinary tract, including cystitis and acute and chronic pyelonephritis, are described in more detail in Chapter 14.

• Other Prenatal Infections

Toxoplasmosis is a protozoan that infects animals as well as people. It seldom produces symptoms in adults, yet antibodies, a sign of past infection, are found in 25 to 45 percent of all women of childbearing age. Your doctor can determine if you've had a recent infection by checking for a significant increase in antibodies in your blood. If the infection occurred before you became pregnant and is dormant, no treatment is required.

One of every 500 to 1,000 babies is born with toxoplasmosis; 20 percent of these infants will have congenital defects. The most serious consequences are mental retardation, brain anomalies, and eye damage. There are no drugs available in the U.S. for treating this infection in pregnancy, since the effective antibiotics are hazardous to the fetus. Spiromycin, which has been used extensively in Canada and France without any evidence of danger in the mother or the baby, is not available here. Toxoplasmosis can be prevented by avoiding raw or undercooked meat (cooking kills the microorganism) and by avoiding contact with the feces of a cat that may be infected.

A pregnant woman who is traveling to a region where an infectious disease such as malaria or amebiasis is endemic should seek her doctor's advice about vaccines and preventive care. Such illnesses can increase the risk of complications for her and her child.

· Sexually Transmitted Infections

The incidence of sexually transmitted diseases has increased dramatically in recent years. A greater number of women of childbearing age are acquiring these infections, thus putting a greater number of unborn children at risk.

Syphilis

Each year there are 100,000 new cases of syphilis reported in the U.S. The thin, corkscrewlike organism that causes syphilis, called a spirochete, thrives in a warm, moist environment. Entering the body through any tiny break in the mucous membranes, the germ burrows its way into the bloodstream. Contaminated needles and sexual contact, primarily intercourse, are virtually the only means of transmission.

Syphilis produces a painless lesion, or chancre, that appears at the site where the spirochete entered the body: mouth, throat, or vagina. This lump may be the size of a dime or smaller. The incubation period, from infection to the appearance of the chancre, ranges from ten to ninety days; three to four weeks is average. Any sexual contact during this time is likely to spread the infection. Since it does not hurt, the chancre may not be noticed at all. With or without treatment, it disappears in three to six weeks. At that stage, the spirochetes enter the bloodstream and begin moving through the body.

Anywhere from one to twelve months after the chancre's appearance, the secondary symptoms of syphilis appear: a skin rash, whitish patches on the mucous membranes of the mouth, temporary baldness, low-grade fever, headache, swollen glands, large moist sores around the mouth or genitals. The symptoms may last for days or months, but eventually they too disappear. During the next stage—the latent phase—the spirochetes attack various organs inside the body, including the heart and brain. For two to four years, there may be recurring infectious and highly contagious lesions on the skin or mucous membranes. But syphilis loses its infectiousness as it progresses. After the first two years, a person rarely transmits syphilis through intercourse; after four years, syphilis is usually not contagious. Until this stage of the disease, however, a pregnant woman can infect her unborn child.

If a fetus is infected early in pregnancy, it may die or be disfigured. If infected later, it may show no signs of infection for months or even years after birth, but the child may then become disabled with the grave symptoms of late syphilis, including heart, brain, and spinal cord damage. Treatment of an infected pregnant woman halts the spread of syphilis to her unborn baby; the drugs used are the same as at other times: penicillin or a similar antibiotic. In forty-five states, prenatal screening tests for syphilis are required in order to detect the disease in an expectant mother.

Babies with congenital syphilis have a 50 percent mortality rate in the perinatal period. Those who survive always have the stigmata of the disease, including healed sores on the skin, an enlarged liver and spleen, inflammation of the eyes, fever, jaundice, disfigured teeth, and bowed legs. More symptoms may develop if the baby is not treated with penicillin immediately after birth.

Gonorrhea

Gonorrhea is one of the most common and dangerous sexually transmitted diseases. In men, the symptoms are painful and obvious, including a burning sensation on urination and thick pus oozing from the penis; but in as many as nine out of ten infected women, there are no symptoms at all. The gonococcus can live undetected in the vagina, cervix, and fallopian tubes for months, even years. Five percent of sexually active American women have positive gonorrhea cultures and are unaware that they are carriers of the disease.

Eventually most women develop complications as the gonococcus spreads through the urinary-genital tract. Gonorrhea can cause a chronic pelvic infection that lasts for years and causes irreversible damage to the reproductive organs. Pelvic inflammatory disease (PID), or salpingitis, is a serious complication that can result in an increased risk of ectopic pregnancy or in sterility.

If a woman with gonorrhea does become pregnant, her disease becomes a threat to her unborn baby, increasing the risk of preterm labor, growth impairment, and neonatal illness. Gonorrhea also can cause a serious form of conjunctivitis, an inflammation of the baby's eye that may lead to blindness. As a preventive step, silver nitrate or antibiotic drugs are placed in the eyes of all newborns after delivery. The infant's external genitalia also may become infected at birth. Treatment for gonorrhea in pregnancy is the same as at other times: penicillin or a similar antibiotic.

Herpes Simplex

Herpes comes from the Greek word meaning "to creep" and denotes one of the most common viral infections in the U.S. Characteristically, herpes causes blisters on the skin or mucous membranes. Once a person has contracted herpes, it never goes away completely, although it may go into long latent periods.

Herpes simplex comes in two varieties: herpes I, which causes cold sores and fever blisters, and herpes II, which causes lesions on the genitals. However, the two forms often mix, and herpes II, the only significant venereal disease proven to be caused by a virus, may appear both in the mouth and on the genitals. There may be as many as 25,000 new cases a year, and it is now considered to be epidemic.

Genital herpes appears as a series of very painful blisters of the vulva (lips of the vagina), cervix, pubic area, buttocks, or thighs. The first blisters persist for two to four weeks and then disappear, recurring for one- to two-week periods, often during times of stress or in response to sunlight. There is no cure for these extremely painful, persistent, and annoying lesions. Drying agents, such as ethanol, applied on the skin may decrease the severity of the discomfort and shorten the duration of the attack.

If you have genital herpes and become pregnant, the greatest risk occurs at delivery, if there are active lesions in your birth canal. The percentage of babies who develop herpes after such exposure is not known, but the consequences for those who do are devastating. The mortality rate for newborns with visible herpes lesions is as high as 60 percent; half of the survivors suffer serious damage to their eyes and nervous system. A cesarean delivery is recommended to bypass the infected area. Vaginal delivery is safe if there are no active lesions; a culture of suspected areas of infection can confirm whether or not active herpes virus is in the reproductive tract. A baby whose mother has active lesions may be kept isolated from other babies to prevent any spread of infection. The mother must follow meticulous washing and hygiene measures to protect her baby.

Chlamydia (Non-Specific or Non-Gonococcal Urethritis)

The most common venereal disease in the U.S. is urethritis, infection of the urinary tract by a bacterium other than gonococcus. In many cases, that bacterium is *Chlamydia trachomatis.* In men, this infection can cause pain during urination and a clear, watery discharge from the penis. In women, there are no apparent symptoms of the infection. If untreated, chlamydia can lead to pelvic inflammatory disease (PID), which may cause scarring of the fallopian tubes and increase the risk of infertility and ectopic pregnancy.

Chlamydia is difficult to diagnose. Although techniques for culturing the bacteria have been developed, they are not readily available at all hospitals. In various studies of pregnant women, chlamydia was diagnosed in 5 to 15 percent. Approximately 30 to 50 percent of their babies were born with conjunctivitis, an eye inflammation that can impair vision, and 10 to 20 percent developed pneumonia. At many hospitals, chlamydia is the major cause of neonatal pneumonia, a potentially deadly problem for the very young. The problem of chlamydia is under extensive investigation at several centers.

Before or after pregnancy, tetracycline is the antibiotic used to combat chlamydia. Because it can impair normal development of a baby's teeth, another antibiotic, erythromycin, is used in pregnancy.

• Prognosis

Researchers are just beginning to unravel the mysteries of infections before and at birth. Only recently have they learned that infections may have subtle as well as devastating, and long-term as well as short-term, effects. Some prenatal infections may cause preterm labor or growth impairment and may play a role in learning and behavioral disorders detected years later.

Sophisticated laboratory procedures, including electron microscopy, immunoelectrophoresis, and radioimmunoassays, are making it possible to diagnose prenatal infections much earlier and much more precisely than in the past. This may permit earlier treatment for the mother and preventive care for her baby. The ultimate goal is to find ways of checking these silent, unseen threats before they can claim or cripple more babies' lives.

17 . *Problems Within the Womb*

IN MOST PREGNANCIES, the intricate, systematic process by which a baby prepares for life goes smoothly. If something does go wrong, it's likely to be only a minor variation from the norm, such as a pregnancy that continues a bit longer than anticipated. In a relatively small percentage of pregnancies, however, more serious complications develop. They can become perplexing medical challenges, for physicians must try to diagnose and treat problems they cannot observe in patients they cannot touch, knowing that the consequences of what they do—or don't do—could have a lifelong impact.

In this chapter we'll look at different sorts of problems that occur before birth: the unique risks of a baby who spends too much time in the womb, the concerns about too much or too little amniotic fluid within the uterus, the dangers related to the placenta's function and abnormalities of the umbilical cord, and the range of defects, some minor and some major, that affect 2 to 4 percent of all newborns.

· Postmaturity: The Overdue Baby

It isn't unusual for your delivery date to come and go without any indication that your baby is preparing to leave your womb. About 8 to 11 percent of pregnancies extend more than two weeks beyond the normal forty-week term. Very often the baby actually *isn't* overdue; the estimated delivery date is inaccurate. As we explained in Chapter 3, "dating" a pregnancy can be difficult, particularly if your menstrual cycles have been irregular, you have been using oral contraceptives, or you couldn't recall the first day of your last period. And if you've had a prolonged pregnancy before, your baby may, like its older sibling, stay longer than usual in the womb.

A postterm pregnancy is not a complication in itself, but it is a reason for increased observation. The incidence of fetal problems and death rises in babies who remain too long in the womb. Some overdue babies can develop a condition called postmaturity, caused by a placenta that no longer can supply adequate nutrients. The baby stops growing or actually begins to lose weight, becoming progressively weaker within the now-hostile environment of the womb. At forty-three weeks, the risks to a baby's life are two to five times higher than at term; at forty-four weeks, they can be as much as seven times higher.

Your doctor will rely on tests of the baby's condition (see Chapter 5) to determine if there is any immediate danger. He or she will weigh the relative risks of continuing the pregnancy. If there is danger to your baby, labor will be induced, and if induction fails, a cesarean delivery will be performed. If tests show that the baby is vigorous and growing, your obstetrician may choose to do nothing until labor begins spontaneously.

· Abnormalities of the Amniotic Fluid

Your unborn baby lives in a watery world; the fluid that protects and surrounds it is a complex substance formed in different ways at different stages of pregnancy. In the first months, much of the amniotic fluid is absorbed from the mother's tissues. Water and other small molecules cross through the amniotic membrane and collect within it. During the second trimester, the developing fetus begins to swallow amniotic fluid and to produce urine. All these processes determine the amount of fluid in the amniotic sac.

The average amount of amniotic fluid in pregnancy is about 2,000 milliliters, the equivalent of 2 quarts. An excessive amount of fluid creates a condition called polyhydramnios or hydramnios. A lower-than-normal amount of fluid is referred to as oligohydramnios. An unborn baby can face increased risk from either a surplus or a deficiency of amniotic fluid.

In as many as 1 of every 60 pregnancies, there is a minor degree of hydramnios. You're likely to have a greater volume of amniotic fluid if you're carrying twins or if you have diabetes or Rh incompatibility problems. Severe hydramnios, with more than 3,000 milliliters of fluid within the amniotic sac, is quite rare. It occurs in about 1 of every 1,000 single-fetus pregnancies. A fetal defect that interferes with swallowing, such as a constriction of the esophagus, can be the cause. Certain neural tube defects, in which spinal cord fluid spills into the amniotic fluid, also can cause extreme hydramnios.

Hydramnios may develop gradually, or its onset may be quite sudden. If you develop this problem, your first symptom may be difficulty in breathing, caused by your enlarged uterus pressing against your diaphragm and lungs. Your obstetrician may not be able to feel the baby by palpating your abdomen or to hear its heart through a stethoscope because of the excessive fluid. Your legs and abdominal wall may be swollen, because your uterus is squeezing the blood vessels, interfering with normal drainage and circulation. Diagnosis is based on a combination of clinical examination and ultrasound.

Minor degrees of hydramnios usually require no treatment. The risk of preterm labor, placental abruption (page 153), and hemorrhage after delivery increases in more severe cases. The doctor may use amniocentesis to withdraw some of the excess fluid, a procedure which may have to be repeated several times. You and your baby will be monitored closely, often in the hospital, for any signs of complications.

Oligohydramnios is a less common problem, although it is equally serious. Sometimes the volume of amniotic fluid falls to just a few milliliters. The baby, unable to float, may be in danger of resting on the umbilical cord, cutting off its supply of oxygen and blood.

Medical scientists don't completely understand the causes of oligohydramnios, though in many instances the problem begins with an obstruction of the baby's urinary tract or a leak in the amniotic membranes. A fetus that never develops kidneys (a rare and fatal birth defect called renal agenesis) will be unable to produce urine and, therefore, will have very little amniotic fluid.

Oligohydramnios early in pregnancy is dangerous because the fetus, with no protective cushion of fluid around it, is subjected to pressure from the mother's organs. It also is at greater risk of abnormal lung development. Later in pregnancy, if the baby's lungs are mature, early delivery may be performed to avoid potential dangers such as compression of the umbilical cord.

· Abnormalities of the Placenta

The placenta is crucial to your baby's development and well-being. Shaped like a large multipartitioned bowl, it weighs about 1½ pounds at birth and contains about 100 milliliters (3 ounces) of blood. Throughout pregnancy the placenta transfers oxygen and molecules of nourishment from your blood to your baby's; waste products pass the other way for disposal by your lungs and kidneys. This process also conveys important immunities from you to your baby that help protect it against potentially harmful microorganisms.

Any disorders that interfere with the placenta's development or its blood supply may increase the risk to the baby. If an adequate supply of blood does not reach a part of the placenta, an area of tissue may die; this is called a placental infarct. This process, associated with the normal "aging" of the placenta during pregnancy, may jeopardize your baby if it occurs before term or if your pregnancy continues long past your due date. The baby may have impaired growth because of placental "insufficiency," or inability to provide proper nourishment.

Placenta Previa

In 1 of every 200 pregnancies, the placenta lies very low in the uterus, rather than on the top or side, and covers the cervix so the baby cannot enter the birth canal. This is called placenta previa—quite literally, "placenta first." The placenta itself is normal; its position is not.

The most frequent symptom is painless vaginal bleeding, usually not occurring until the last trimester. Ultrasound confirms the diagnosis. The greatest immediate danger to the baby is preterm birth. Your doctor may put you on bed rest in order to prevent a too-early delivery and to gain more time for your baby's development. If you continue to lose blood, you may be hospitalized and watched closely. If bleeding continues, either episodically or persistently, you may require transfusions to maintain your blood volume or, if blood loss is severe, early delivery.

If placenta previa occurs very late in pregnancy, the primary risk shifts from the fetus to you. Blood transfusions may help to restore normal blood volume, but if the bleeding cannot be controlled and your blood pressure falls too low, there is a risk that you will go into shock. To prevent this danger, your doctor may deliver the baby immediately, usually by cesarean section. If only a small part of the cervix is covered by the placenta—a very rare occurrence—a vaginal delivery may be possible.

Placental Abruption

In one of every fifty to eighty pregnancies, a portion or all of the placenta separates from the uterine wall before, rather than after, delivery. Sometimes the separation is partial; sometimes it is complete, leading to the death of the baby and increasing the risk of hemorrhage in the mother.

The primary cause for placental abruption isn't known, but it is more likely to occur if you have hypertension, smoke heavily, or had a similar problem in a previous pregnancy. The first symptoms are usually vaginal bleeding and abdominal pain, varying from mild to "knifelike" and extremely severe, beginning in the second half of pregnancy. Ultrasound confirms the separation of the placenta.

If the placenta has not separated completely, your doctor may take a conservative wait-and-see approach, allowing the pregnancy to continue in order to avoid the risks of premature birth. The major danger to the baby is a cutoff of its oxygen supply. If the placenta separates completely, only delivery within minutes can save the baby's life.

Placental abruption also endangers the mother, because of the possibility of such problems as shock, blood-clotting abnormalities, and failing kidney function. Hospitalization and immediate care, including blood transfusions and intravenous fluids, may be necessary to maintain normal blood volume. The method of delivery—vaginal or cesarean—depends on the extent of the separation, the mother's condition, and the existence of any other complications.

· The Umbilical Cord

Umbilical cords vary dramatically in length. Some perfectly normal cords are 18 centimeters (7 inches) long; others are 120 centimeters (47 inches). Boy babies have slightly longer cords than girl babies, for unknown reasons. The cord usually reaches its full length by the twenty-eighth week.

A normal umbilical cord has two arteries that carry blood to the baby. If there is only one artery, there is an increased risk of fetal malformations, miscarriage, and a baby who is small for gestational age. Sometimes the flow of blood is cut off, usually by twisting or compression. The baby may kick vigorously to free the cord, alerting its mother to the potential danger.

Many parents worry about the hazard of a cord being wrapped around the baby's neck during delivery. This is not an uncommon occurrence—it happens in about 17 percent of births—but it is not particularly threatening. Usually the obstetrician simply slips the still-slack cord over the baby's head.

· Birth Defects

The vast majority of babies are born healthy and perfect in every way. Anomalies, or malformations, occur in only 2 to 4 percent of newborns. Most congenital defects are minor and can be corrected easily after birth. The most common are club foot, polydactyly (extra finger or toe), cleft lip or palate, hip malformation, and imperforate anus (a rectum that ends in a blind pouch). None of these problems causes permanent damage, and with proper treatment a baby with any of these defects can grow up to live a full, normal life.

Yet even though the odds are overwhelmingly in their favor, all parents worry about having a baby with a defect that might claim or cripple its life. Some fear that they might pass on a genetic defect (see Chapter 4). Others wonder if the baby's development might go awry at some step along the way.

In the past, parents had to live with such fears until the day of delivery. It was impossible to know whether the baby hidden within the womb was normal or deformed. Today, by means of sophisticated prenatal diagnostic tests (described in Chapter 5), it is possible to detect many—but not all—serious abnormalities.

At this time the ability to diagnose problems before birth far outstrips perinatologists' ability to correct them. Certain prenatal treatments—such as intrauterine transfusions of red blood cells for babies with Rh disease and injections or corticosteroids to accelerate lung maturation before a preterm delivery—have helped save thousands of babies. In experimental operations, perinatologists are attempting to correct certain birth defects before delivery. They have proven that surgery on an unborn baby is possible, but much more experience and time for follow-up are needed to determine if such prenatal therapy can prevent impairment in babies with specific defects.

At this time only three birth defects—and only certain types of these—seem likely candidates for such pioneering operations: hydronephrosis (a urinary tract obstruction), diaphragmatic hernia (a defect in which the intestine pushes through the diaphragm wall, interfering with normal lung development), and hydrocephalus (the buildup of excessive fluid within the skull). All three are rare anomalies that have devastating effects when they do occur.

Even if there is no prenatal treatment for a defect diagnosed before birth, foreknowledge can alert physicians to the potential danger. If, for example, an ultrasound scan shows that the baby's intestines have developed in a sac outside the abdomen—an anomaly called an omphalocele—surgeons can prepare to begin operating to replace the intestine within the baby's abdomen minutes after delivery. The prognosis for babies who receive such quick treatment is excellent.

Prenatal diagnosis can lift a heavy burden of fear for many parents. If a grave defect, such as anencephaly (lack of normal brain development) or agenesis (lack of kidneys), is detected, they might choose to terminate the pregnancy rather than continue and give birth to a doomed child. But in most cases the results of prenatal tests are negative, and parents are able to await the birth of their child with anticipation rather than apprehension.

18 . *Doubling Up: Twins*

TWINS ARE UNUSUAL but not rare; they occur in approximately one of every eighty pregnancies. Most twins develop normally in the womb and are healthy at birth. However, a twin pregnancy increases the possibility that the babies might encounter problems. Because of that risk, doctors pay special attention to a woman carrying more than one fetus. After all, three lives are at stake under circumstances more complex than usual.

If you are expecting twins, you can expect some differences in the way your body changes and in the recommendations you are given about taking the best possible care of yourself and your babies. In this chapter we'll describe how twins develop, how to find out if you're carrying twins, what risks to consider, and what to expect throughout pregnancy and delivery.

· How Twins Are Formed

A twin pregnancy may be the result of the fertilization of one or of two eggs. For reasons that are not well understood, a fertilized egg sometimes divides into two, and each identical half of the original egg develops into a twin. Such twins are called monozygotic (one-egg), or identical. They are always of the same sex and have exactly the same genetic makeup, so they will develop and look very much alike. Identical twins occur in about 1 of every 250 births and are considered an "accident" of nature, unrelated to hereditary patterns of twinning or to the mother's age or race.

If two eggs are released at the same time and fertilized by two different sperms, two genetically distinct individuals will develop. They are described as dizygotic, or fraternal, twins. Two thirds of all twins are fraternal. In the United States, 1 of every 70 black women has fraternal twins, compared to 1 out of every 100 white women. The highest incidence of fraternal twinning in the world is in Nigeria, where twins occur in 1 of every 45 pregnancies. In one rural Nigerian community, a set of twins is born in every 22 pregnancies. The lowest incidence of twins—about 4 per 1,000 births—occurs in China and Japan.

Older women, particularly between the ages of 35 and 39, are more likely to have fraternal twins. Mothers of twins generally tend to be more fertile and to have borne more children than the average. According to statistics, the chance of having twins increases with the number of children already conceived.

Heredity also plays a role in the formation of fraternal twins. You are more likely to bear twins if your mother was a fraternal twin; the tendency toward twinning does not seem to be passed on by fathers. The likelihood of twins also increases if you've been taking hormones to treat an infertility problem. One fertility drug, Clomid, has been linked to a twin conception rate of 60 to 80 per 1,000 births.

The placenta and membranes that protect and surround twins are formed during the first weeks in the womb. Sometimes twins share a single gestational sac and placenta; sometimes each twin is enclosed in a separate sac and is nourished by a separate placenta. The risks of certain complications, such as poor growth, are related to whether your twins are sharing—and possibly competing for—the nourishment a single placenta provides.

· Are You Carrying Twins? How to Find Out

It's not unusual for any mother contemplating her enlarging belly to wonder if there is more than one baby within her womb. Particularly in a first pregnancy, you may think that only twins could account for your astounding new shape. Some of the clues of twin pregnancy may indeed be right before your eyes: You should be suspicious if you are gaining weight more rapidly than usual and if your abdomen is growing at what may seem an alarming rate. Later in pregnancy, you will be able to see and touch various parts of both babies' bodies through your skin. You also may feel kicks and movements all over your abdomen, rather than just in one particular area.

Your doctor will look for clues in your blood. The characteristic hormones of pregnancy—human chorionic gonadotropin, alpha fetal protein, and human placental lactogen—are typically at higher than normal pregnancy levels in a woman carrying twins. But since elevated levels of some of these hormones may indicate other problems affecting a single baby, these measurements don't provide absolute proof. Your doctor also will check your fundal height (the distance from the top of your uterus to your pubic bone); this measurement will increase more quickly than usual if there is more than one fetus in your uterus.

After the eighth week, a sensitive ultrasonic stethoscope may be able to pick up two heartbeats. However, sometimes the sound of one baby's heart muffles the sound of the other. If you haven't been getting regular checkups or if your weight gain and growth have not been unusual, several months may pass before you or your doctor suspects a twin pregnancy. Often twins aren't detected until the final trimester.

The definitive method of diagnosis is ultrasound, which confirms the presence of more than one fetus, pinpoints their location in the womb, and provides information about their approximate age and size.

· What to Expect

A twin pregnancy is a variation from a single-baby pregnancy, but not necessarily a dramatic one. If this is your first pregnancy, every sensation may be new and unfamiliar. If you've already had a single-fetus pregnancy, you may view the differences in your size or general comfort as primarily a matter of degree.

Your body changes just as any other expectant mother's does, but those changes may be more marked because of the greater needs of two babies. Your blood volume increases as much as 50 to 60 percent over prepregnancy levels. Your uterus becomes much larger than in a single pregnancy; by term the combined weight of your uterus and the two babies may be 15 to 20 pounds. The total volume of fluid within your amniotic membranes also is greater, and the weight of the placenta, if shared by your twins, is larger.

Because of these changes, you may be more susceptible to the various discomforts of pregnancy. As your enlarging uterus presses against other organs, you may experience heartburn and indigestion. You may feel as if you can't breathe often or deeply enough, even though you will be taking in more oxygen than you did before you were pregnant. You may have to urinate much more frequently, and your legs and feet may swell after you've been on your feet for only a brief time. These are common conditions; many can be prevented or minimized by following the advice given in the chart in Chapter 3. Regular moderate exercise can help you feel better, but you should check with your doctor before beginning any strenuous activities. If you're feeling very fatigued, you may be advised to schedule one or two rest periods during the day.

You can prevent many serious problems for yourself and your babies with good prenatal care and nutrition. In order to meet the needs of three bodies—yours and your twins'—it is essential to eat well-balanced meals with an increased amount of protein, carbohydrates, and folic acid. Your weight gain may be 12 to 13 pounds more than the usual 24 to 27 pounds for a single pregnancy. If your nutrition and weight gain are good, your babies are much less likely to have low birth weights. By taking a daily iron supplement as recommended by your doctor, you can avoid another common problem in twin pregnancies—anemia, a deficiency of oxygen-carrying red blood cells in your body.

You may need to restrict your activity more in the final weeks of pregnancy either because of the risk of preterm labor or because of your now-considerable bulk. Various tests may be performed to indicate how your babies are faring (see Chapter 5). Your doctor also will check their positions in your womb, because this may determine whether you will have a vaginal or cesarean delivery. About 75 percent of twins both have their heads downward in the womb in the typical "vertex" position. However, almost any combination of positions is possible: one twin may be vertex and the other breech (foot first); both may be breech; one may be vertex and the other lying across it in a transverse position.

· Risks to Your Babies: What to Consider

The fact that you conceive twins doesn't mean that you will have more problems, but obviously it does increase the potential for complications.

Preterm Labor

While twin pregnancies account for only 1 percent of all births, they are associated with 10 percent of perinatal deaths. A primary reason for these losses is prematurity: as many as half of all twin pregnancies end in premature deliveries (see Chapter 9). Obstetricians have noted that the more babies in the uterus, the shorter the duration of pregnancy. An average single-baby gestation lasts forty weeks; a twin pregnancy, thirty-seven to thirty-eight weeks; a triplet pregnancy, thirty-five weeks. For reasons that are not fully understood twins and triplets are less likely to get the time they need to complete their development.

You can help. As described in Chapter 9, there are early warning signals of preterm labor, and you should learn how to monitor yourself for "silent" contractions in the second half of your pregnancy. If you detect the telltale symptoms of preterm labor, seek immediate treatment. If labor has not progressed too far, there is an excellent chance that your uterine contractions can be controlled by means of drugs that relax the uterus. Your doctor may recommend some preventive measures to buy your babies more time in the womb, including increased bed rest and restrictions on your activity around and outside the house. Premature twins are vulnerable to the same problems as other babies who enter the world too soon, but in general they are more likely to survive than single babies born at the same early age.

Growth Problems

Twins typically do not grow to the same size or at the same rate as single babies, and identical twins tend to be smaller than fraternal ones. The average birth weight for 40 to 60 percent of twins is less than 2,500 grams (5½ pounds). And twins, like other small-for-gestational-age infants, may encounter big problems if they start off life too tiny (see Chapter 8).

Your nutrition and weight gain during pregnancy are critical in assuring proper nourishment for your babies. However, other factors can also play a role in their growth before birth. For example, if your twins share a placenta and amniotic sac, they are in greater competition for nourishment, and one or both may have impaired growth. In about 1 of every 1,000 such instances, one twin will receive a greater share of nutrients and develop a much larger blood volume than normal. Such "twin-twin transfusions" can result in the birth of one very small baby and one very big one. The large infant is likely to look much healthier, but it often is the one at greater risk. With an excessive amount of blood, low blood pressure, and a tiny heart, the bigger baby may develop heart failure and circulation disorders. These often prove to be fatal. The smaller baby encounters the same difficulties as any other SGA infant.

Birth Defects

These are uncommon in all pregnancies, single or multiple, but there have been reports of a slightly increased incidence of anomalies in twins. The most frequent problems are club foot, polydactyly (extra digits), heart abnormalities, and neural tube defects (see page 36). Some of these problems may occur if there is a delay in the splitting that takes place when a single egg divides to form identical twins. This may explain why identical twins seem to be at somewhat greater risk of birth defects than fraternal ones. All twins face the same genetic risks as other babies, but prenatal testing may be more difficult because of the need to test two fetuses and possibly two amniotic sacs.

Hydramnios

A single baby usually floats in about 2 quarts (2,000 milliliters) of fluid within the amniotic sac; two babies sharing the same sac need more fluid in order to float and move freely before birth. It is not unusual for there to be a larger volume of amniotic fluid, but occasionally there can be an excessive amount. This condition, called hydramnios or polyhydramnios, is described in more detail on page 151.

Maternal Complications

As in every pregnancy, your well-being has an all-important impact on your baby's health and development. Any chronic medical problems, such as diabetes or epilepsy, or any complications that develop during pregnancy such as pre-eclampsia (which is more frequent in twin mothers), can jeopardize the babies. Very often good preventive care can eliminate the risks or minimize the effects of an illness. Because of the increased demands of a twin pregnancy, you may be especially likely to develop gestational hypertension (see Chapter 11) or gestational diabetes (see Chapter 13). Frequent checkups can detect these problems before they become serious threats to your babies.

Stillbirths

Twins are two to four times more likely to die before birth than single infants, possibly because of the increased risks associated with growth impairment, birth defects, and such maternal complications as hypertension and pre-eclampsia. In the first half of pregnancy, there is a greater risk of miscarriage; if only one twin dies, the other is in jeopardy. The risk of its also dying is exceedingly high if both babies shared the same amniotic sac, because their umbilical cords may be intertwined. The various tests of an unborn baby's well-being described in Chapter 5 may be used to check on your twins' condition in the last trimester.

· Double Delivery

It's impossible to predict exactly what will happen at any birth, and doubly difficult to anticipate every potential circumstance in a twin delivery. That is one reason why obstetricians disagree about the best and safest approach to twin births.

The pattern of labor and delivery for a twin birth is generally the same as for a single-fetus pregnancy (see Chapter 20). Usually the larger twin is the first to exit from the womb, followed within minutes by the second baby. If the bigger twin is in a breech position, or if the smaller one is the first to move down the birth canal, delivery may be complicated.

Some obstetricians feel that cesarean delivery is better for all twins. Others feel that cesareans are necessary only under certain circumstances, such as breech presentation or excessive delay after the delivery of the first twin. Your doctor will base his or her decision on your twins' gestational age, size, and well-being, along with their position in your womb and any obstetrical complications that may occur in the course of labor. With good medical care, mothers of twins are not more likely to develop problems during or after delivery. However, the experience may seem doubly intense and exhausting—though it also can be twice as exhilarating.

19 . *The Longest Months: Coping with a Complicated Pregnancy*

FOR WOMEN AT RISK, pregnancy may seem like the best of times and the worst of times. One day you may be so excited about becoming a mother that you can feel yourself beaming. On another day you may be almost overwhelmed by anxiety about something going wrong. Every pregnant woman knows what it's like to live through such roller-coaster experiences, with higher highs and lower lows than at any other time of life. You may have all the normal highs and lows and joys and worries—and experience them far more intensely.

Pregnancy always is a life crisis—although usually a positive one—that affects your emotions as profoundly as it changes your body. What goes on inside your mind is complex and varied, just like what is happening within your womb. During this time you may change the way you think about yourself, your partner, and your future. At times, coping with those changes and the feelings they produce may seem more difficult than handling the physical aspects of your pregnancy. That is why it may help to stand back and get a more objective perspective on your feelings. In this chapter we'll try to provide that sort of view by considering the psychological impact of a complicated pregnancy, the common feelings of women at risk, the way some women handle the emotional challenges, and the role the father can play before his baby is born.

· What It Means to Be at Risk

You probably expected to have a textbook pregnancy, just like the ones you read about or like the experiences of your sisters or friends. Your first reaction to discovering that you're at risk may be surprise. Yes, you expected your life to change—but later rather than sooner. In a complicated pregnancy, however, you may have to start making adjustments long before you even see your baby.

A major difference between a low-risk pregnancy and a complicated one is a matter of time. You may think your entire life has come to revolve around your medical care. You may have checkups scheduled every week or every other week. Diagnostic tests for you and your baby can take up additional time. If you're diabetic, you'll spend more and more time monitoring your blood sugar levels and adjusting your insulin doses. If you have a pre-eclampsia or other medical complications, you may have to collect twenty-four-hour urine samples periodically or undergo frequent blood tests. If your baby is in increased jeopardy, you may spend up to two hours every day monitoring its movements for any indication of danger.

Many women react to this situation with conflicting emotions. They appreciate the careful attention and conscientious treatment that may help save their babies, but they resent the extra demands. They may feel that they're sacrificing their own life to an unremitting process with an uncertain outcome. If they were ambivalent about becoming pregnant in the first place, the complications may heighten their misgivings. And, of course, they're apprehensive—afraid for their babies and perhaps for themselves too.

Your own reaction can depend on the problem that put you at risk. If you have a chronic illness, such as systemic lupus erythematosus or diabetes, you may have thought and talked about potential problems in pregnancy long before you conceived. Because of your illness, you may be accustomed to making adjustments in your lifestyle and to seeing a great deal of your doctor. But if you've never had any medical problems, complications that develop in pregnancy, such as gestational hypertension or Rh incompatibility, may be very unsettling. You can find yourself spending more time in a doctor's office or hospital than ever before in your life. Some necessary diagnostic tests and procedures can be intimidating and uncomfortable. For the first time in your life, you may have to face painful realities such as the possibility of having a sick baby or of losing your baby before or after birth. At times you may feel more like a patient than an expectant mother.

Such reactions can be intensified if you have to be hospitalized during pregnancy, perhaps because of preterm labor or a flare-up of a chronic kidney disease. Hospitalization always is difficult. The hospital routine can seem alien; you may be unable to sleep because of the incessant noise and the regular checks on your condition. Worry about your baby and the forced separation from your family can add to your anxiety.

If you are taking drugs—to lower your blood pressure or to fight an infection, for instance—you may worry about their potential effects on your baby. You also may experience side effects that can be minor or extremely uncomfortable. Added to such immediate concerns is the question of money. There are extra costs involved in your care, and you and your partner may wonder whether your insurance will cover the additional expenses of a high-risk pregnancy or any special care for your baby after birth.

As your delivery date approaches, you'll be exceptionally eager for the long months of pregnancy to end, but you also may be anxious about problems during or after delivery. If there is a chance that you or your baby will need additional care, you may be transferred to a perinatal center with special facilities. It can be very upsetting to leave behind familiar faces and a familiar setting, particularly when you are already feeling vulnerable.

Yet even though such stressful situations provoke anxiety, you should keep in mind that most aspects of your pregnancy *are* normal. Your baby is following the same timetable of preparation for life as other babies. Your body is changing in the ways that every expectant mother's does. Even the emotions you're feeling have been experienced by countless mothers-to-be over countless years of time. Being at risk does add certain elements to your pregnancy, including a need for more precautions, more surveillance, and more technology. Understanding what is happening within and around you can help, but some of the essential excitement of creating a new life may indeed be diminished.

· Common Feelings

You may think that you're the only pregnant woman who's grown frustrated during the months of waiting, or who's gotten inexplicably angry with her husband or doctor, or who's thought to herself, "This kid had better be worth all I'm going through." You're not.

Every pregnant woman—regardless whether the pregnancy is wanted or unwanted, low-risk or high-risk—has some negative feelings about herself, her baby, and the people around her. These emotions are normal. They don't mean that you won't be a good mother. They simply reflect a strain that could fray anyone's nerves.

One of the characteristics of pregnancy is emotional variability, which is called "lability" in medical terminology. You can be laughing one minute and burst into tears five minutes later. A minor run-in with a rude salesclerk or an impatient driver can lead to anguish or rage. Many pregnant women are so unnerved by their emotional reactions to trivial matters that they wonder if they're becoming unbalanced. Actually, psychiatric disorders in pregnancy are rare. What you're feeling is a normal response: your moods are reflecting the rapid changes within you and the adjustments you have to make to the world around you.

All pregnant women have moments, or hours, or days of depression or anxiety. For many, each trimester brings new emotional challenges along with its physiological changes. If you're at risk, you'll feel the same flood of new emotions: anxiety and anticipation, fear and excitement, doubt and commitment. But you may find yourself burdened with other feelings as well.

One of the most common is guilt. You may automatically assume that you are responsible for the problems in your pregnancy and blame yourself for complications that have absolutely nothing to do with you or your behavior. Many women try to find the one "terrible" thing that they did to cause their hypertension or preterm labor or the baby's growth impairment. Perhaps it was that glass of champagne, the skiing vacation, the Mexican food. This sort of thinking is an attempt to make sense out of a difficult situation. It is easier to focus on one cause for your problem—however illogical—than to feel completely out of control.

The best way to handle feelings of guilt or inadequacy is to find out more about what really is happening to you and your baby. Almost always, your fantasies are worse than the realities. Talk to the doctors and nurses about your pregnancy. Ask questions about your treatment. If you're intimidated by high technology, find out how ultrasound or electronic monitors work. If you're worried about a drug's effects, discuss the possible risks. You have a right to ask such questions and get straightforward answers. It's *your* health and *your* baby that are at stake.

Some women insist that they don't want to know about risks and problems. That's not an unusual attitude; it's a way of running away from unknown and scary dangers. Yet the more you *don't* know, the more you'll worry and speculate. As you acquire information and understand more, you'll feel less like a patient and more like a participant. You'll be more in control and less plagued by groundless fears. One woman in preterm labor, for example, overheard conversations about her baby's lungs and assumed that her baby had no lungs and was doomed. She spent hours in panic until she learned that the doctors' concern was about lung maturity and that her baby had a very good chance of surviving. You also might ask your doctor about the psychological effects of any of the drugs you're taking. It's not unusual for some medications to affect your mood swings or to cause a temporary depression. Understanding their influence can help you cope with the emotional impact.

Even though most complicated pregnancies have happy endings, you may find yourself worrying that your baby will die or be disfigured or handicapped. No one will be able to give you any absolute guarantees, but you can find out what the risks really are. Because so many serious threats to your baby can be prevented by proper care before birth, you also may gain new motivation for taking extra precautions.

· Coping

Pregnancy is never a good time to audition for the role of Superwoman. Even if you're accustomed to being independent, you're likely to find the support of your friends and family more important now than before. Psychiatrists have noted that emotional support can play a key role in the outcome of a pregnancy.

Two mothers-to-be may develop the same complications, and their babies may face similar medical risks. Almost always the woman who has a strong support system fares better, and so does her baby. A mother who's alone or isolated from family and friends is at greater risk even if a minor problem develops, while a woman with a supportive partner may have a successful pregnancy despite multiple risks. At some hospitals women who've experienced high-risk pregnancies or perinatal losses have organized support groups. It can be enormously comforting for you to talk to women who know exactly what you're going through.

It's important that you express your feelings. You may feel that negative emotions like anger or depression will reflect poorly on your ability as a future mother. Yet simply ventilating these feelings can defuse their intensity. When a psychiatrist analyzed the emotional needs of a group of high-risk mothers hospitalized during pregnancy, he found that very few needed professional counseling. What helped these women most was a genuine appreciation for what they were experiencing and honest information about what was happening to them and their babies.

Sometimes the most difficult thing you are asked to do for your baby is nothing at all. It's not unusual for a doctor to prescribe bed rest if you're at risk of preterm labor or have a heart or blood pressure disorder. And whether you're at home or in the hospital, you may chafe under the restrictions on your activity. It helps to keep a diary, or to cross passing weeks off on a calendar. Some women catch up on reading; others take up a craft, such as quilting. If you have other children, it may become essential to have help with household chores and with their care. Often a spouse or relative can pitch in around the house, while friends can help with shopping and cooking.

Try to take care of as many details related to your pregnancy as far in advance as possible. If you have a chronic illness and are planning a pregnancy, check your insurance in advance to make sure you'll be fully covered. You may want to find out where the nearest perinatal center is, and talk to your obstetrician about arranging a transfer if special care is needed. Many hospitals have social workers who can help mothers-to-be cope with practical details if they are hospitalized or confined to bed during their pregnancies.

Given all the stresses of a complicated pregnancy it is probably more surprising that most women cope so well than that they occasionally feel discouraged or worried. One reason is motivation. Everything you go through in your pregnancy, including the extra care and precautions, is a step toward the goal of having a healthy baby. Some women talk about "the carrot at the end of the stick." Others simply say that they feel that the time and effort required before their babies are born will pay off afterward. "I can put up with anything for nine months," said one woman, "especially when I know that these months may change the rest of my life."

· The Father's Role

In the past fathers often had little more than a walk-on role in a pregnancy. However, in the last decade the father has become a featured participant, particularly in the labor and delivery rooms. In a complicated pregnancy, he can play a crucial role long before his child's birth. His support, encouragement, and commitment to his mate and their unborn child can be critical factors in overcoming risks before birth.

Even in a normal pregnancy, a father may feel ambivalence and some jealousy of his mate's preoccupation with herself and their unborn baby. A high-risk pregnancy forces the father-to-be to confront the same fears and doubts as the expectant mother. He may feel greater pressure to help his wife and baby. Occasionally the burden of increased responsibility seems too great, and a man will run away—if only for an evening. Others turn away emotionally, distancing themselves from their wives. One reason is their sense of helplessness and sometimes of neglect. One man described the constant attention that everyone gave his wife during her pregnancy and added plaintively, "No one ever even asked me how *I* was doing."

Fathers, as well as mothers, may find it easier to cope with the stresses of a problem pregnancy if they understand what is going on and why. Men who accompany their partners to the doctor's office can ask questions and find out what they can do to help. Often the father can become an active participant in the pregnancy—helping a diabetic woman monitor and record her blood sugar levels, practicing breathing exercises if his wife is on bed rest, attending classes on childbirth preparation.

A high-risk pregnancy brings some couples closer than ever, while others are pulled apart. Usually a couple responds to the challenges in ways that are characteristic of their relationship. Some may feel that their unborn baby—the "fruit of our union," as one mother put—is a symbol for their marriage: if the baby is at risk, so is their relationship. Others feel a stronger commitment to each other than ever before: in a sense, they are proving their love for each other as they provide mutual support in a time of immense stress.

PART 3

The Critical Hours

20 . *From Womb to World: Labor and Delivery*

EVER SINCE SHE FIRST suspected she was pregnant, Maryann Branley thought about the inevitable climax to the months of waiting: the birth of her baby. With each passing week, her feelings about delivery changed, swinging from anticipation to apprehension, from curiosity to impatience. Reading books about labor and delivery, she stared in wonder at the photographs of women giving birth and tried to imagine the way she might feel and act.

When Maryann talked to her mother about childbirth, she was struck by the differences that a single generation had made in medicine's and mothers' approaches to delivery. When she was born, delivering a baby was considered something a doctor did. Her mother had been semiconscious throughout the process; her father had been exiled to a waiting room down the hall. As she made plans for her own baby's arrival, Maryann discovered an almost bewildering array of options for birth settings, attendants, and preparatory classes. What appealed to her most was the concept of family-centered childbirth, for she felt that Mark's constant presence and support would be reassuring through the long process of labor and delivery.

Like Maryann, you may want to learn as much as you can about the process by which a baby journeys from womb to world, so you can participate as fully as possible. In this chapter we'll describe Maryann's labor and delivery and discuss both the norms and exceptions of the process of giving birth.

· Normal Labor and Delivery

Maryann's body began preparing for labor and delivery in the last weeks of her pregnancy. As is common in a first pregnancy, she felt a lightening in her final month and found it easier to breathe deeply.

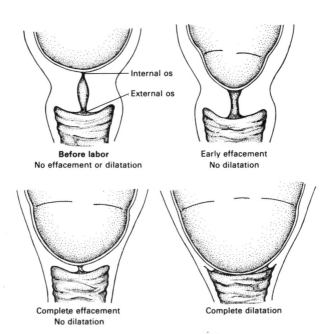

Internal os

External os

Before labor
No effacement or dilatation

Early effacement
No dilatation

Complete effacement
No dilatation

Complete dilatation

(from Reeder, Mastroianni, and Martin, Maternity Nursing, *14th ed. J. B. Lippincott, 1980)*

The pressure on her diaphragm eased because her baby's head had settled into her pelvis, much like an egg resting in an egg cup. The baby moved less vigorously than before, but Maryann often felt jabs from its feet and arms. The "engagement" of the head increased the pressure on her bladder, and she had to urinate more frequently. She also began to feel some unfamiliar sensations in her lower abdomen and perineum, the area around the opening of the vagina. Her obstetrician explained that these brief, irregular contractions, called Braxton Hicks contractions, were not a sign of true labor. Occasionally she'd feel a different buzzing sort of sensation as her baby's head pressed against the muscles of her perineum. When she noticed a small plug of mucus, tinged with drops of blood, that had been discharged from her vagina, she realized that labor probably would begin soon. This gelatinous material had sealed the opening of the uterus from the vagina throughout the months of pregnancy.

Maryann was not at all aware of some other changes taking place within her body. Her cervix, the narrow canal between the uterus and the vagina, gradually "ripened," or softened, and was transformed into a flat opening in the bottom of her womb; this process is called effacement. In first-time mothers like Maryann, these changes take place over several days; in women who've already borne children, they may occur in a period of a few hours. They are the necessary preliminaries to labor and delivery.

True labor is divided into three stages. In the first and longest stage, the cervix dilates, or opens, completely to a width of 10 centimeters (4 inches). In the second stage, the baby moves through the birth canal and emerges from the vagina. The third stage consists of the delivery of the placenta, sometimes called the afterbirth. The initial part of first-stage labor, the latent phase, is a time of relatively gradual cervical dilation, usually to a width of 3 or 4 centimeters. First-time mothers spend an average of 8 hours in the latent phase; in women with previous deliveries, the mean duration is 5.3 hours.

Maryann realized labor would begin soon when she felt a sudden gush of fluid from her vagina; her amniotic membranes had burst. Within a few hours her contractions intensified, lasting longer and occurring more often. She kept a careful record of the intervals between contractions and of their duration and called her obstetrician when they were five minutes apart. As she and Mark drove to the hospital, she used the breathing techniques she'd learned in childbirth preparation class to cope with the pain. She knew that the relaxation techniques were important, since anxiety could prolong the duration of the latent phase beyond the normal upper limit of about twelve to eighteen hours for a first delivery.

At the hospital, her obstetrician recorded her rate of dilation and the time she'd been in labor. Maryann's labor followed the normal S-shaped labor curve for the first stage: her latent phase lasted about nine hours. When she was dilated to 4 centimeters, the active phase began. Frequent checks showed that she was dilating at a rate of about 1 centimeter an hour, with contractions occurring every two or three minutes and lasting for sixty to ninety seconds.

As Maryann's cervix was dilating, her baby was beginning its de-

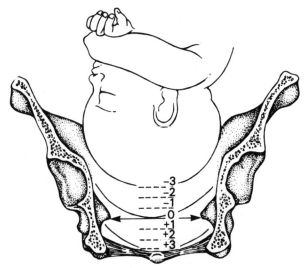

"Stations" indicate the baby's position as it moves through the birth canal *(from Reeder, Mastroianni, and Martin, Maternity Nursing, 14th ed. J. B. Lippincott, 1980)*

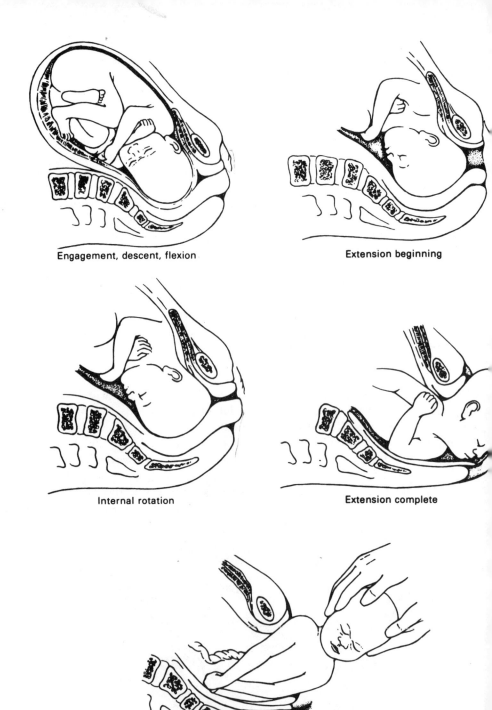

Engagement, descent, flexion

Extension beginning

Internal rotation

Extension complete

Expulsion

The process of being born *(from Reeder, Mastroianni, and Martin,* Maternity Nursing, *14th ed. J. B. Lippincott, 1980)*

scent. The obstetrician noted its progress by marking its "station," or location, in her birth canal. As the drawing on page 175 illustrates, a baby is at a station of −3 when its head or presenting part is just below the mother's pelvic inlet. When the head moves into the inlet, the baby is at 0 (zero) station; at the lower part of the pelvis, it is at +1. Maryann's baby was at +1/+2 station when, after four hours of active labor, her cervix had dilated to 10 centimeters.

Maryann began to feel an overwhelming urge to push as the second stage of her labor began. Coached by her husband and a maternity nurse, she tried to work with the forces within her body to press her baby through the birth canal. After about forty-five minutes, her baby's head crowned, or became visible. Because of the likelihood of some tearing of her vagina and the muscles below, her obstetrician performed an episiotomy, an incision from the lower end of the vagina toward the anus. The episiotomy would need fewer stitches and heal more easily than an irregular tear.

Like most babies, Maryann's infant emerged gradually—first the head, then one shoulder, then the other, then the rest of the body. In a matter of seconds the newborn boy took his first breath. The obstetrician clamped the umbilical cord and lifted him onto Maryann's stomach. As the new parents introduced themselves to their son, the third stage of labor proceeded. Maryann's uterus became firmer. The baby began to suck at Maryann's breast, stimulating the production of oxytocin, a hormone that triggers contractions. The contractions compressed the blood vessels in the uterus, reducing blood loss. Within five minutes, the placenta was expelled from Maryann's vagina. Her obstetrician inspected it, examined her uterus to make sure that none of the products of the pregnancy remained inside, and sutured her episiotomy. The process that had begun some 280 days before was complete: Matthew Branley was born.

· Special Deliveries

Like Maryann's, most births are uncomplicated and require little, if any, medical intervention. A great many of the women considered to be at risk throughout pregnancy have normal labors and deliveries. However, complications can arise—whether or not there have been problems in pregnancy—and they may develop suddenly. Often quick treatment is necessary to minimize the risks to mother and baby. The more you know about special circumstances and problems during labor and delivery, the more you'll understand about what is happening to you and your baby.

Spontaneous Rupture of the Membranes

The amniotic membranes usually rupture, or burst, during labor. In about 10 percent of pregnancies, they break beforehand. If your membranes rupture before your thirty-sixth week, you should seek immediate care for a possible preterm delivery. After the thirty-sixth week, according to statistics, 70 percent of women begin labor within twelve hours of rupture of their membranes; another 15 percent within twenty-four hours; another 10 percent by seventy-two hours. Because of the risk of infection, labor usually is induced in the remaining five percent.

There is increased risk of infection of the amniotic sac after rupture of the membranes. This problem, called chorioamnionitis, can endanger you and your baby before and after delivery. The symptoms of infection include fever, abdominal pain and cramping, a drop in your blood pressure, and uterine tenderness. Amniocentesis may be used to confirm an infection if you are not yet at or near term. If the membranes rupture in a full-term pregnancy and labor does not begin spontaneously within twelve to thirty-six hours, it is induced to avoid the significant risks associated with perinatal infection.

Induction/Augmentation of Labor

Your baby may be at increased jeopardy in the womb for a variety of reasons, including growth impairment, postmaturity, or Rh incompatibility. Your doctor may induce labor, either by amniotomy (artificial rupture of the membranes) or by intravenous administration of a drug that stimulates uterine contractions. Usually induction cannot be attempted unless your cervix has begun to soften and thin.

Amniotomy stimulates labor by releasing the fluids from the amniotic sac, which leads to stronger contractions of the uterus. As with spontaneous rupture of the membranes, there is increased risk of infection if labor does not begin within twelve to seventy-two hours. The other method of induction is the use of a synthetic form of a hormone, oxytocin, which causes the uterine contractions. Oxytocin initially is infused into the blood stream in low doses, which gradually are increased to produce stronger contractions that simulate labor. Both the mother and baby must be monitored carefully by the nurse or physician because of the chance that the contractions could become too frequent. Once a good pattern of contractions is established, the oxytocin often can be reduced or even stopped, and labor proceeds naturally.

Occasionally oxytocin is used to augment contractions if the first stage of labor is abnormally long. Administered in the same way as for induction, oxytocin speeds up or intensifies the contractions to avoid the risks associated with extended delays in labor.

Abnormal Labor Patterns

Your obstetrician will evaluate your rate of dilation during the latent and active phases of labor to determine if either phase is unusually prolonged. Lack of normal progress in the latent phase may be the result of anxiety, oversedation, or weak, ineffective contractions. The same factors can cause a delay or slowdown in the active phase. Occasionally a baby is unable to move into the birth canal because of its size, a condition called cephalo-pelvic disproportion, or its position. Your obstetrician may initiate electronic fetal monitoring (page 52) to check on your baby's condition and may recommend augmentation of your contractions with oxytocin because the risks to the baby increase if labor is abnormally slow. In cases of cephalo-pelvic disproportion, a cesarean delivery may be the only option.

Abnormal Presentation

About 5 percent of babies travel down the birth canal in a position other than top-of-the-head-first. In about 3.5 percent of births, the bottom part of the baby's body—either its buttocks or its feet—is at the lower part of the uterus; this is called a breech presentation. More rarely the baby lies horizontally in the womb in a transverse position.

If your baby is in a breech position by your thirty-sixth week, your obstetrician may try to turn it around in utero by a procedure called version. With slow, gentle pressure, the baby's head is slowly turned downward. Version can be successful in preventing a breech birth, but some babies return to a foot-first position soon afterward.

Delivery of a breech baby may be more complicated, because the lower body is less effective as a "wedge" in pushing through the birth canal and its head could be caught in the pelvis. Some obstetricians feel that vaginal delivery is safe if the baby is not unusually large and labor proceeds normally, but spoonlike instruments called forceps may be necessary to support and protect the baby's head. A newborn specialist generally stands by at delivery in case the newborn is suffering from hypoxia (oxygen deprivation) and needs help breathing.

A cesarean birth is sometimes considered safer for a breech baby if it is unusually large (more than 8 pounds); if its head is hyperextended (angled away from the body); if it is premature; if labor has been prolonged; if one foot is dangling in front of the other; if the mother's pelvis is narrow or unusually shaped; if there have been medical complications during pregnancy; or if the mother has had a previous breech delivery that resulted in perinatal death or damage. While a cesarean involves fewer risks to the baby than a vaginal delivery requiring the use of forceps high in the birth canal, it does not eliminate all the dangers associated with a breech presentation. Abdominal delivery of a breech baby is more complicated than one of a baby in vertex (head-down) position.

Forceps Delivery

Forceps are metal devices that come in a variety of shapes and sizes. They are carved to dovetail into each other so they cannot exert too much pressure on a baby's head. Low, or outlet, forceps are used to protect a baby's head and guide it through the lower birth canal. They are most often used to prevent damage during vaginal delivery of a premature or small-for-gestational-age baby or if the birth process is prolonged. Mid forceps are used primarily if the second stage is prolonged and the baby shows signs of distress. High forceps, inserted into the upper birth canal, are no longer used because a cesarean delivery is considered safer for the baby. The primary risks associated with forceps are damage to the baby, such as "molding" of the head, as a result of incorrect application, and lacerations (cuts) of the soft tissues of the mother's vagina and perineum.

Vacuum Extraction

A vacuum extractor consists of a metal or plastic cap that is attached to the unborn baby's head, a suction pump, and a tube connecting the two. As the mother pushes down in the second stage of labor, the obstetrician pulls on the tube, controlling the amount of suction so the force is strong enough to speed up the baby's progress but not so strong that it harms the baby. Obstetricians use this technique for the same reasons they might employ forceps, primarily to accelerate the birth of a baby in jeopardy after a prolonged second stage. Vacuum extractions can be used only if the baby is in a head-first position. Its risks include cuts of the baby's scalp, sometimes with formation of a blood clot under the scalp, and cuts or tears of the mother's soft tissues. Doctors choose this technique instead of forceps largely because of personal preference.

Cesarean Birth

A cesarean birth involves an operation, performed under general or regional anesthesia, in which an incision is made through the abdomen and uterus and the baby is lifted out of the womb. Until the twentieth century, the risks of operating were so great that such deliveries were extremely rare. As recently as two decades ago, cesareans were performed only when there was clear danger to the mother's survival, and accounted for about 2 to 5 percent of all births. Now more than 10 percent of all births are cesareans; at some hospitals the cesarean rate is higher than 20 percent. Many obstetricians feel that this method of delivery is safer than labor and vaginal delivery for the most vulnerable babies, including those that are small for gestational age, premature, twins, or in a breech position.

There is considerable controversy over the issue of whether too many cesareans are performed. National committees made up of obstetricians, health policy experts, and consumers have established guidelines on appropriate indications for a cesarean delivery. According to their recommendations, a cesarean is considered the safest option for delivery in *some* instances of: placenta previa or placental abruption; Rh incompatibility with signs of acute fetal distress; maternal complications such as hypertension, pre-eclampsia, or kidney disease; severe growth impairment; active herpes simplex lesions in the birth canal; postmaturity; and prolapse of the umbilical cord (a problem in which the cord slips in front of the body, and vaginal delivery can cause compression of the cord and a cutting off of the baby's oxygen and blood supply).

Depending on individual circumstances, a cesarean *may* be indicated if there is: a breech presentation, an abnormal labor pattern, a failure of induction following rupture of the membranes, fetal distress, or cephalo-pelvic (head-pelvis) disproportion (which may be the result of the size of the baby's head or the mother's pelvis or a failure of the force of the contractions).

If you have had a previous cesarean birth, you may be able to deliver vaginally the next time; but the decision on the safest type of delivery for you and your baby will depend on the type of uterine incision used in your first cesarean and on whether the same risk factors, such as cephalo-pelvic disproportion, develop again during labor and delivery. If the previous uterine incision was low and transverse (across the uterus), the risk of rupture during normal labor and vaginal delivery is about 0.5 percent. If the incision was vertical, the risk can be as high as 10 percent, which is considered too dangerous to allow normal labor and vaginal delivery.

The most commonly used incision today is low and transverse. However, if speed is essential or the placenta is in an unusual position, the obstetrician may use a classical vertical incision on the top of the uterus. A low-flap vertical incision, which is made on the lower part of the uterus but runs up and down so the incision can be enlarged quickly if necessary, is sometimes used for premature babies in an unusual position (such as transverse) and for some twins.

The type of skin incision used to open your abdomen does not affect future deliveries. Most obstetricians make a "bikini cut" right below the pubic hairline.

Like other operations, a cesarean delivery requires surgical preparation, including shaving of the abdomen and upper pubic hair. Either general or regional anesthesia may be used, and a catheter is inserted into the bladder to drain off urine. With a regional anesthetic, the mother is awake but numb from the waist down, and at many hospitals the father can remain with her to provide emotional support.

Once the abdomen and uterus are open, the amniotic sac is punctured, and the fluid is suctioned. The obstetrician reaches under the baby and lifts it from the womb. Usually the time from the first cut to delivery is only four or five minutes. It is the repair of the incisions on the uterus and abdomen that takes much longer.

Parents who plan and prepare for a vaginal delivery may be disappointed if a cesarean becomes necessary, but the more you know about a cesarean birth, particularly before delivery, the more easily you may understand the need for it. Some mothers report a spectrum of negative emotions after a cesarean, including disappointment, helplessness, guilt, and depression. The subsequent physical discomforts—including the pain, nausea, and abdominal gas that are common after any abdominal surgery—may contribute to the sense of unhappiness. There

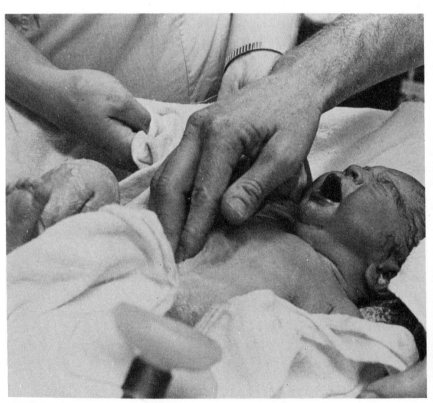

A life begins (Stanford University)

are somewhat increased risks, primarily of infection and blood clots. (To prevent clotting you should begin walking the day after delivery.) The typical hospital stay after a cesarean is five to seven days, and you should refrain from strenuous activities, particularly heavy lifting, for several weeks.

· Postscript

A baby is born. And in their delight and amazement most parents remember not a sequence of orderly stages, but a blur of physical and emotional experiences unlike any they've ever known before.

Maryann Branley recalls the hard work of the first stage, with Mark guiding her through well-practiced relaxation techniques, massaging her back, repeating words of love and encouragement. There were moments when she thought the contractions would never end, yet afterward it seemed hard to believe that almost an entire day had passed. The pain was real and intense, yet strangely acceptable. And when Maryann talks about her labor and delivery, she speaks most of the excitement, mounting throughout the second stage and culminating in her first view of her new son and the sound of his wailing. She cried. Mark cried. Only little Matthew, 8½ pounds, 21 inches long, and perfectly healthy, seemed calm as he lay in Maryann's arms, looking around at the big, bright new world he'd just entered.

21 . Special Care for You and Your Baby: Perinatal and Neonatal Centers

"THAT'S IT! That's it! Good. Almost there. I can see the baby's scalp. Now push again. Come on, give it all you've got!"

The obstetrician and nurses join in the chorus, their eyes focused on the bulging, glistening tissues around the opening of the woman's vagina. The baby's head emerges, and the obstetrician's hands guide it into the world. First one shoulder, then the other appears. The rest of the body slips out quicky. There is a sudden silence. The baby is an odd shade of very pale blue.

From the corner of the delivery room, two surgically masked and gowned figures rush over. In a flurry of rapid motions, the cord is clamped and the baby placed in their hands. They carry the baby to a heated, lighted table. It lies limp as they place a tube into its windpipe and pump air into its lungs. For what feels like an eternity the room is quiet: everyone is listening, waiting for the reassuring sound of the baby's first cry. Finally the baby trembles, coughing and whimpering. The nurses smile and, for the first time, look into the mother's face. She is crying softly. "Is my baby all right? Is it going to live?" Only after hearing the first feeble wails does she ask if it's a boy or a girl.

It is a girl, and she's not out of danger yet. But her chances for surviving and growing up healthy are far better than they might have been, primarily because of where she was born—at a perinatal center fully staffed and equipped to give her and her mother the extra care they both needed during the critical period before, during, and after birth.

Throughout this woman's pregnancy, her obstetrician had been concerned about her chronic kidney problems, especially after she developed hypertension and signs of pre-eclampsia. She was initially hospitalized for a few days at the community hospital in her small hometown in western Nevada. But the obstetrician felt that she and her baby would be much safer if she was transferred to a perinatal center several hundred miles away. There she would be assured of immediate access to experts in perinatology and other specialties and to the special equipment critical in caring for her and her baby.

A small plane, specially designed to serve as a flying ambulance for mothers and babies, transported her to the perinatal center, where she was examined by a perinatologist and a specialist in kidney diseases. Her baby's condition was evaluated by sophisticated diagnostic tests. When the perinatologists felt that both she and her baby were in increasing danger, they induced labor, and the neonatologists (doctors specially trained in the care of the newborn) were called in for the delivery.

Now, lying back on the delivery table moments after giving birth, the new mother stares anxiously at the table across the room where her baby lies, hidden by the cluster of doctors and nurses bending over its tiny form. She waits as they make sure the baby's airway is clear, her heart rate strong, her blood pressure and volume normal. Before transferring the baby to the intensive-care nursery—along with her heated bed, oxygen supply, and entourage of attendants—they pause to introduce the baby to her mother. "Don't worry," the neonatologist says with a reassuring smile. "We're going to take very good care of her."

Taking good care of babies at risk at the very beginning of their lives has been one of the greatest challenges to modern medicine. Research into the beginnings of life was the first step. Pioneering methods of diagnosis and treatment were the next. But the ultimate key to saving babies before they're born is making sure that the best perinatal services are available to the mothers and babies who need them most. That is why perinatal centers have been set up across the country. They are the hubs for regional networks made up of obstetricians, pediatricians, geneticists, nutritionists, radiologists, nurses, transport teams, and local hospital staffs.

Perinatal centers are, in essence, minihospitals designed for unborn and newborn patients and their mothers. Usually part of major medical centers, they provide "tertiary," or highly specialized, care for those at greatest risk during the perinatal period. They are equipped with state-of-the-art technology to diagnose and treat problems and are staffed twenty-four hours a day by doctors and nurses experienced in overcoming risks and handling emergencies before, at, or after delivery.

In this chapter we will provide an introduction to perinatal centers, describing the people you're likely to meet and the equipment you're likely to see if you or your baby require extra care. We'll also discuss some of the special issues facing mothers of babies at risk, including bonding, breast-feeding, and taking the baby home.

· What to Expect

You aren't likely to go to a perinatal center for your first prenatal visit unless your obstetrician is on its staff or you live in the neighborhood. Most women are referred to a center by their obstetricians, for reasons that include many of the problem described in this book. Though your doctor may have considerable expertise in handling complications of pregnancy, he or she may still feel that you will benefit if diagnostic facilities or consultants in other specialties are immediately available. You may continue under your own doctor's care, going to the center periodically only for special tests; or you may become a regular patient of an obstetrician specializing in high-risk pregnancies and go to the center for regular checkups. Some women at risk are transferred to a perinatal center shortly before their babies' birth because the womb is a far safer transport system than any incubator. Occasionally a complication develops suddenly, late in an otherwise normal pregnancy, and the obstetrician decides that the mother and her baby should be at a perinatal center.

Who's Who

At most perinatal centers, you and your unborn baby will be cared for by perinatologists, obstetricians who have special training in maternal-fetal medicine and high-risk pregnancies. After delivery, neonatologists, pediatricians who specialize in treating newborns in their first days and weeks of life, will care for your baby.

Your "attending" physician—the doctor who admits you, delivers your baby, and assumes primary responsibility for your care—will be an obstetrician. Depending on your needs and circumstances, specialists in other fields, such as cardiology or neurology, may examine you and consult with your doctor about your care. Many perinatal centers have teaching programs for fellows, residents, and medical students. Fellows are fully trained obstetricians or pediatricians who are acquiring additional training in either perinatology or neonatology. Residents are recent medical-school graduates who are completing their postgraduate training in obstetrics or pediatrics. The fellows and residents, sometimes called house officers, may be closely involved with your own and your baby's day-to-day care and may be present at your delivery. During labor and delivery, an anesthesiologist (a physician whose specialty is anesthesia) will administer whatever analgesics (pain-relieving drugs) or anesthesia is needed.

Nurses with special training in perinatology or neonatology will provide continuous care to you and your baby. Throughout pregnancy, nurses may provide valuable advice and support in caring for yourself and your baby. Some centers have nurses who specialize in working

with high-risk mothers. During labor, a nurse will monitor your progress, check on your baby's condition, and oversee the administration of
medications. One or two nurses will assist at delivery. If your baby
requires intensive care after birth, a nurse assigned only to him or her
will provide round-the-clock treatment and monitoring. As the baby's
condition improves, less intensive nursing care is needed, and one nurse
may care for two or three other infants as well as your baby.

In some situations, other health professionals, such as genetic counselors and nutritionists, may become involved in your care. At many perinatal centers, social workers are available to help parents cope with
necessary arrangements for hospital care, home visits by a nurse, or
financial assistance.

What's What

Medical technology plays an important role in perinatology, for it extends the staff's diagnostic and clinical skills. Many of the highly sophisticated machines serve as electronic eyes and ears that alert the
medical team to the earliest signs of a problem. The equipment used
for diagnosis before birth and for monitoring your baby's condition
during labor is described in Chapter 5. You may find this technology
more reassuring than intimidating if you understand how it works and
why it is used.

If it's possible that your baby will need extra care after birth, try to
visit the intensive-care nursery at the perinatal center *before* delivery.
More technology is concentrated in this area than almost anywhere else
in a hospital, except perhaps the operating rooms, and a first visit can
be an overwhelming experience. At any time of day or night, the nursery is usually bustling with activity. Lights blink. Alarms buzz. Doctors
and nurses huddle over incubators containing doll-sized babies. Wear-
ing only diapers so they can be observed and treated easily, the infants
seem almost hidden by wires, tubes, and bandages. If you learn before
delivery what the machines are and what they do, you'll find it easier
to concentrate on your baby afterward.

· The Tiniest Patients

Most babies are healthy from the moment they arrive in the world.
About 10 percent are at risk because of problems that developed before
or during birth, and approximately 25 percent of these—nearly 3 of
every 100 babies—are high-risk infants requiring immediate intensive
care. They are often so vulnerable that they need round-the-clock
treatment and a special environment that only very sophisticated technology can provide. More than 600 nurseries—many at perinatal centers—have been set up around the country to give these babies the

extra care that can save their lives or prevent permanent impairment.

The intensive-care nursery mimics the world within the womb. An optimum temperature is maintained by means of "warmer beds," or incubators, and heat and moisture are kept at levels that prevent stress on your baby's fragile metabolism. If your baby has breathing problems, a carefully controlled amount of oxygen may be provided through a small round plastic hood over its head. Occasionally air is pumped directly into the baby's lungs by means of an endotracheal tube placed into its mouth and down its windpipe. Fluids and medications may be given to the baby through a catheter (hollow tube) inserted into the main blood vessel of its umbilicus. Other blood vessels, particularly those on the scalp, may be tapped to serve as supply lines for nutrition. Small metal and paper discs, connected to monitors of heart rate and respiration, are safety measures that let the doctors and nurses know if there is a change in the baby's vital signs or if the medical devices malfunction.

Many of the babies in any intensive-care nursery were born prematurely. Some of the problems they face are described in Chapter 9. Others spent a full term in the womb but are small and fragile at birth; their risks are discussed in Chapter 8. Babies who develop Rh incompatibility disorders may need immediate treatment at birth and during their first days in the world; Chapter 10 provides information on their needs. The infants of diabetic mothers may require careful monitoring as their metabolism adjusts to life outside the womb (Chapter 13); the babies of women with other chronic illnesses also may require special attention (Chapter 15). Infection is a threat that may begin before, during, or after delivery; its effects can range from mild to lethal (Chapter 16). Babies who stay in the womb too long and develop postmaturity problems and those with congenital defects sometimes require intensive care (Chapter 17). While their medical problems may be quite different, all of these babies are alike in one important respect: they are fighting for a chance to live.

· Special Issues for Mothers of Babies at Risk

Bonding

Bonding is defined as the formation of a unique relationship that endures through time. It is very much like falling in love—a developing, deepening, enriching experience that binds two people together. Many mothers say they sense a growing bond with their babies before birth, as they feel their movements within the womb. In the best possible circumstances, the bonding of both parents with their new child begins in their shared experience at birth. The mother and father of a healthy, full-term baby are able to touch, hold, and kiss their infant, to respond to cries and coos, to relate to their new son or daughter face-to-face and skin-to-skin.

In less-than-ideal situations—if the baby is premature or sick, if the delivery is a cesarean, if the mother develops medical complications—the process of bonding may seem more difficult. The image of the new family caught up in a transcendent experience at birth has been popularized so extensively that many parents feel that anything less is at best a disappointment, and at worst a failure. They also worry that if they don't have immediate contact with their child, they may never form a durable bond.

Psychiatrists assure parents of babies at risk that they need not worry that the "glue" of family bonds will set and dry by any particular time after birth. If your baby needs intensive care, you will be encouraged to visit as often as you want. Despite the incubators, wires, and alarms of the intensive-care nursery, you can make physical and emotional contact. Many nurseries have round-the-clock visiting hours. As soon as your baby is strong enough, you can take him or her from the incubator to hold, rock, feed, diaper, and bathe.

The Parents' Vigil

Most parents are stunned when their newborn baby is whisked away to an intensive-care nursery. Months of anticipation culminate in a bewildering combination of joy at the baby's arrival and fear for its survival. There is no typical response, no right or wrong feelings. It's not unusual to feel nothing other than the normal exhaustion that follows labor and delivery.

But all too soon the new parents have to confront the heartbreaking possibility that their baby may not survive. Their fears may intensify if they do not get clear information on the baby's condition or if the baby is taken to a distant hospital. The father may feel torn between staying at his wife's side or accompanying the baby to the nursery.

Some parents are disappointed if their baby doesn't look like the chubby infants of television commercials—and high-risk babies often don't. One mother of a baby born three months prematurely thought he looked like a monkey. "I wondered how I could ever love a baby like that. Then I started stroking his chest with my finger. I noticed that his nose was a little like mine and his ears were definitely the same shape as my husband's. Pretty soon I was thinking, 'God, how could I *not* love this baby?' "

Some couples immediately assume the worst and experience anticipatory grief, mourning even though the baby is still alive. Others cling to any shred of hope, any possibility that the baby will recover. Both reactions have very little to do with the actual severity of the infant's problems and more with the parents' style of responding to a crisis.

The longer the baby is in danger, the longer the parents ride the roller coaster of hope and fear. The initial sense of panic often gives way to denial and disbelief. The parents may question the actions and competence of the staff, search for other opinions and options, and resist any change in treatment plans.

"I found myself shouting at one of the nurses one day, and then I realized that actually I was jealous of her," one mother recalls. "She was doing a better job taking care of my baby than I could. I resented that. And I was afraid that my little boy would become more attached to her than to me."

The staff nurses and doctors may themselves feel the strain of prolonged uncertainty about a baby's fate. Unless they develop an effective way of communicating, the parents may feel that the staff is indifferent to their wishes or is keeping information about their baby from them. Caught up in surges of anger, fear, sadness, and despair, the parents may lash out at the doctors or nurses—or at each other. "The hardest thing to accept is the helplessness," says a neonatal nurse. "That's what really gets to the parents. They want to do something, and they can't. They want us to do something, and we can't. The frustration eats at them."

As a baby faces each crisis and survives, hope flourishes. The initial symptoms of anticipatory grief—crying, sleeplessness, irritability, loss of appetite—gradually ease. Waves of depression and fear may return, but less frequently and less intensely. As the parents spend more time with the baby and acquire more information from the staff and from other parents with similar experiences, they begin to make realistic plans for the future. They may seek advice on coping with any long-term problems the baby may have or on adapting to those problems.

It's impossible not to worry when your own baby's life hangs in the balance. But there are ways to cope with the waiting and the worry. One of the best is talking, particularly with parents who've gone through the same experience. At many nurseries, parents have formed support groups, often organized by a social worker or volunteer. A mother whose own baby had been in intensive care calls or visits the parents of a baby newly admitted to the nursery. Unlike even the most well-meaning friends or relatives, she understands what the couple is feeling; she's been through it all herself. "It was so good to be able to talk to someone who understood, really understood, and who'd survived," says one mother. "It made me feel that I wasn't alone."

Another boost for the spirits is learning about babies who once were as small or as sick as your newborn and who now are growing up healthy and normal. Some nurseries keep scrapbooks of their "graduates" with "before" and "after" photographs. "My baby looked a lot bigger and stronger than a lot of the preemies in the pictures," says one new mother. "When I saw what sturdy toddlers those sick little infants had grown into, I started thinking about how our little boy would look at his first birthday. It gave me something to look forward to."

Breast-Feeding

Human breast milk is the perfect food for a baby. Breast-fed infants have fewer illnesses and hospitalizations. When they do get sick, they recover more quickly, and their mortality rate is lower. When you breast-feed your baby, you provide more than good nourishment; you pass along protective antibodies that prevent many illnesses in the first months of life. Colostrum, the watery fluid initially produced before breast milk itself appears, is particularly rich in antibodies to protect your baby. The shared intimacy of nursing also strengthens the bond between you and your baby.

Most women who've had complicated pregnancies can breast-feed afterward. If you had a blood pressure disorder, your baby may be very small and unable to nurse immediately, but in the interim you can pump your breasts. The milk is given to your baby through a tube, though there may be a brief period when your milk will not be used because of certain medications you may be taking to lower your blood pressure.

If you are diabetic or developed gestational diabetes, you should be able to breast-feed, but you will have to monitor your blood sugar levels and insulin requirements carefully because of metabolic changes after delivery. With appropriate care, you should be able to control your diabetes by diet alone if you did so before your pregnancy. If you are insulin-dependent, you may have to increase your caloric intake and adjust your insulin doses, as indicated by monitoring the level of sugar and ketones in your blood and urine. You'll have to make further adjustments when weaning your baby. In some women, nursing leads to a temporary remission of their diabetes.

If you've had a cesarean delivery, breast-feeding usually is possible if your baby is healthy. Depending on the type of anesthesia used, you may begin to nurse within twelve hours of delivery, through you may need help from the nurses so you can hold your baby comfortably without disturbing an IV line or catheter. Any pain medications will be administered immediately *after* you nurse, so their levels in your body will have peaked and fallen before your next feeding.

If you develop an infection after a cesarean delivery, you may have to discontinue nursing temporarily, depending on the nature and location of the infection. The most frequent infections in new mothers involve the urinary tract and do not present a risk to the baby. Your doctor will select a medication that will be safe for your baby.

If you developed a cytomegalovirus infection (see Chapter 6) in your last trimester or shortly after delivery, your baby may have a "silent" infection. It's not clear whether or not a newborn can catch this virus from the mother, but breast-feeding generally is considered safe. Nursing actually may be beneficial because her infant may receive protective antibodies from the mother. If you have active herpes simplex lesions at the time of delivery, your physician will assess your condition to determine if there is any risk in breast-feeding.

Low-birth-weight infants may not be able to suck or swallow, although they sometimes can be given breast milk through a tube. For some very sick babies, even tube feedings are withheld for a few days. But even if your baby faces several weeks or months of intensive care, it may be possible for you to maintain your milk supply.

If your baby was postmature, early breast-feeding can help his or her metabolic control. Postmature infants often feed poorly initially and need considerable prodding to suckle. However, once they begin regular nursing, they usually do well and catch up on normal growth. Infants who develop self-limited acute illnesses, such as fever, respiratory infections, colds, or diarrhea, usually do best if breast-feeding is continued. The mother's antibodies may limit the severity of the disease, and nursing itself may provide comfort as well as nutrition.

Babies with certain congenital defects present special problems. Any malformation of the nose, mouth, or jaw, such as a cleft lip or palate, may hinder breast-feeding, and the mother may have to pump her breasts to produce milk that will be given to the baby by tube or dropper. Infants with other surgically correctable defects may not be able to begin nursing until they have undergone surgery. Sometimes breast milk can be frozen and stored to await their recovery. Some mothers whose babies have life-threatening defects choose to breast-feed simply for the close contact with their baby; others decide not to for fear that nursing will only add to their grief if the baby does not survive.

Homecoming

The day you and your baby leave a perinatal center or neonatal nursery can be a milestone in both your lives. All first-time parents feel a bit unsure of themselves as they leave the hospital with their newborn. If you or your baby has been at risk, you may feel particularly wary.

Many parents of babies who were in intensive care fear that they will be incompetent caretakers. Usually it's possible to ease into your responsibilities slowly, starting before your baby is discharged. At first you may feel awkward or tense, fearful of dislodging any tubes or setting off an alarm whenever you pick up your baby. But gradually you'll feel more comfortable changing your baby's diaper or doing simple caretaking chores. Some hospitals have facilities for mothers to spend the final night of their baby's stay there. The mothers take over all responsibility for the baby, but know they have immediate backup and assistance from the medical staff. Once home it's not unusual to feel apprehensive for a while, even if your baby has been given a clean bill of health. But this will pass, and you'll become more relaxed about meeting your baby's needs once you have established a daily routine.

· Prognosis

There is good reason to be optimistic about the future of babies born at risk. For years researchers have been following such babies as they grow, comparing them at various ages to infants who were born healthy. The results of these studies have been encouraging: the vast majority are developing normally—in mind and in body. One psychologist has found that the IQs of these babies at ages 1 and 2 have been improving steadily—under increasingly effective neonatal care—since 1971, when neonatology first emerged as a medical subspecialty.

The brightest outlook is for babies who weigh at least 1,500 grams (3.3 pounds) at birth. Babies who weigh less, whether premature or small for their gestational age, encounter more immediate and more long-term difficulties. Yet even among these tiniest newborns, the number of healthy survivors is increasing. According to one recent study, of the 39,000 babies with birth weights of less than 1,000 grams born each year, 19,000 now survive without any impairment at all.

Neonatologists emphasize that often it is impossible to predict which babies will do well and which will not. Sometimes the effects of problems before birth don't become apparent for years or perhaps decades. And sometimes a baby that seems to have everything going against it— its size, its gestational age, its lung maturity, its feeding difficulties— defies all the odds and grows up not only a survivor, but a winner.

22 . *Unlived Lives: If the Baby Dies*

ON THE UPPER SHELF in the guest-room closet is a photo album with the words "My Life Story" on a bright yellow cover. Nora Daniels bought it when she was five months pregnant. She'd imagined the photos that would cover its pages—pictures of a pink-cheeked, big-eyed, perfect baby and of herself and Paul glowing with a joy greater than any they'd ever known.

Almost two years after Nora bought the album, it holds but a single photograph of Jason Daniels—in his fifth and final day of life. Nora's hands tremble as she opens the album; her voice quivers. The pain of the dream-turned-nightmare still stings. "I was so stunned when the doctors told us that Jason had a fatal heart defect. My very worst fears were coming true. Every mother worries that something awful might happen and her baby might die, but you always think it can't happen to you. It's always somebody else's tragedy."

For the vast majority of mothers, secret fears never do become cruel realities. Most babies are absolutely healthy at birth and the few born at risk generally overcome their initial difficulties and grow up normal and strong. The infant mortality rate in the U.S. today is lower than ever before in our history. Yet some births end in heartbreaking deaths, and every year thousands of couples like Nora and Paul Daniels must cope with the loss of a child they loved but never knew.

According to recent estimates, there are about 20,000 stillbirths and 36,000 deaths (out of more than 3,500,000 births) during or shortly after delivery each year. But the numbers cannot tell the story of what such losses mean to the woman who carried a life within her, the man who fathered her child, and the brothers and sisters, grandfathers and grandmothers, and uncles and aunts who eagerly awaited its birth. In this chapter we'll discuss some of the common experiences of families when a baby dies.

· The Parents' Experience

Like Paul and Nora, most parents are shocked to learn that their baby is dead or dying. It is almost incomprehensible. "I remember hearing the words. The doctor was speaking very slowly and carefully. But the meaning didn't sink in," recalls one woman. "Then the nurse came over to squeeze my hand, and I saw that she was crying. That's when it suddenly hit me that something was wrong, terribly wrong, with my baby."

Some women suspect a possible problem before delivery, perhaps because they've begun to bleed or can't detect any fetal movements. They may hope against hope that their suspicions are wrong. Or they may begin to grieve even before the baby is born. One woman with a chronic disease that increased the risks to her baby worried that every unfamiliar sensation was an ominous sign. "It was a way of protecting myself," she explains. "It was the kind of magical thinking little kids do: If I force myself to think of the scariest thing in the world, then it couldn't hurt me. I constantly jumped to the worst possible conclusion. I'd wake my husband up in the night and say, 'I think the baby's dead.' I didn't want it to be true; I just wanted to prepare myself just in case."

Yet there never is any painless way of facing a baby's death. You might think that the bonds between parent and child grow stronger with time, so that—at least in theory—the death of a toddler or school-age child would be harder to bear. But neither love nor grief are matters of degree. From the moment they realize that they've conceived a child, a man and a woman begin to think like parents. They choose names. They speculate about the unborn baby's hair color or features. They make plans and fantasize. The child-to-be becomes larger than life, the embodiment of their most cherished dreams. If the baby dies, the dreams die too. "It's not like losing a person with a certain identity in your mind," says one mother. "You grieve for the baby you never knew and for the child—the beautiful, perfect, wondrous child—who might have been."

Some women actually feel closest to a child when it is growing within their bodies. Mother and baby share flesh and blood; they react to each other's movements; they affect each other in profound and subtle ways. Every mother "separates" her self from her baby at a different time of pregnancy. Some begin to think of the fetus as a distinct individual when they first feel its kicks; others when they start to "show"; others not until delivery. "If a baby dies late in a pregnancy, the mother may feel that part of her has died," comments a psychologist. "She feels both vulnerable and responsible, as if she did something to cause the loss or should have done something to prevent it."

Very often the mother, blaming herself for the baby's death, tries to track down the specific cause: too much food or too little; working or not working; exercising or not. "I desperately wanted to know exactly what had gone wrong," one woman says, "because I felt that then I could make sure it didn't happen again." Yet it's rare for the doctors to be able to pinpoint the precise problem—and even rarer for anything the mother ate, drank, did, or didn't do to be at fault. In their grief and depression, some women assume the worst about themselves and worry that the baby died because of their own unworthiness. A woman who'd been ambivalent about pregnancy wondered if her doubts played some role. Another, who'd been promiscuous as a teenager, felt that she was somehow morally unfit to become a mother. Such senseless self-inflicted guilt can linger long after the baby's death, gnawing at self-esteem and confidence.

Fathers suffer too, but their pain often goes unrecognized and underestimated. During pregnancy they see themselves as onlookers. If a problem develops, they fear for their wives as well as their unborn children. More than anything else, they feel helpless. "I felt irrelevant," says one man. "There wasn't a thing I could do for the baby, so I focused on my wife. I wanted to be as supportive as I could, even though I really couldn't comfort her. I didn't know the words to say so I'd just hold her and tell her I loved her."

Like mothers, fathers feel guilty. Maybe they shouldn't have traveled so much. Maybe they should have helped out more around the house. Maybe they should have gone to the obstetrician's office more often. As attention focuses on the mother and the ill baby, they also feel left out. One man, frustrated and confused when a deeply wanted baby was stillborn, found himself turning away from his wife. "I was running away, I guess. I'd stay at the office longer. I'd go on trips I could have skipped. I'd drink more than usual. I hadn't been able to save the baby, and I wasn't able to console my wife. She thought I was blaming her. It took a long time for us to work through our individual feelings and reach out to help each other."

Some husbands mask their grief. "She carried the baby, so she was attached to it. I wasn't," they explain. It's not uncommon for the father's grief to remain hidden for several months. Then, as the mother comes to terms with the loss and her need for comfort lessens, he may confront the pain of the baby's death.

Often this is the first loss either parent has experienced, and they may not realize that mourning is a slow process that cannot be rushed. "I've seen couples drift farther and farther apart as they grieve," observes a counselor. "But I've also seen marriages become better than before. Most couples have a characteristic way of dealing with a crisis.

If they can express their feelings and love for each other, they can cope better with such a terrible tragedy."

· Saying Good-bye

Whether the baby is stillborn, dies shortly after delivery, or lives for several weeks before dying in an intensive-care nursery, the parents need to say good-bye. It is not an easy process. In the blur of unanticipated events and shocking news, parents often feel confused and overwhelmed. How did it happen? Why did it happen? Was there any hope? The past and present seem so complicated that it's hard even to think of what to do next. Asked if they want to see the baby, or have a photograph, or cut off a lock of hair, the anguished mother and father may not know what to do.

"I just wanted to hold the baby," one mother remembers. "I'd carried it inside me for nine months, and I wanted to see it and touch it and feel it in my arms. The doctors and nurses had been trying everything to save it. When they told me it was hopeless, I asked for the baby. They sort of hesitated, so I said, 'What could it hurt now?' She died in my arms. At least I have that memory."

If a baby is born with severe birth defects, the medical workers may hesitate to show it to the parents. "My own experience is that it's better for the parents to see the baby," says one counselor. "Sometimes they look at the malformations and realize that the death was a blessing in disguise." One couple learned late in pregnancy that their baby would be born without a brain, a uniformly fatal defect called anencephaly, and would survive for only a few hours. They talked to the doctors and psychologists and decided that they wanted to be with the baby the entire time. After delivery, the nurses wrapped the baby in blankets, covering its deformed skull, and gave it to the parents, who focused on the features that were normal. Afterward they told a counselor that their own fantasies had been much worse than the way the baby actually looked. If a baby's appearance is normal, parents often take comfort in the fact that they have produced an attractive child.

Some hospitals routinely photograph all of the babies who die. If months or even years later, parents want some way of remembering, these photos can be a comfort. A picture, a lock of hair, even a name— all help focus the parent's grief. "Lots of parents feel this vague sense of loss, but it's hard to mourn," says a social worker at a perinatal center. "It helps to have a sense of the real person who died."

Difficult as it may be to face such a decision at a time of deep grief, parents should remember that an autopsy can provide important information that could influence their plans for future children. And because parents so often feel that they are to blame, an autopsy may lift the burden of guilt. Even if it doesn't reveal one conclusive cause of death, very often it can confirm that nothing the parents did was at fault and information from the autopsy may help other babies facing the same dangers.

Some hospitals encourage parents to attend a "death conference" several weeks after the baby's death. The parents meet with the physician who cared for the baby, the primary nurse, and a social worker or counselor. When Paul and Nora Daniels went to a conference about their baby's death, they asked the questions all parents do: Why did our baby die? Did we do anything to cause his death? Will it happen again if we have another baby?

They learned that Jason, who'd looked absolutely perfect at birth, had a heart that was anything but perfect. Because of a malformation very early in its development, his heart could not function and keep him alive. Since fetal circulation is entirely different and doesn't require the same sort of work from the heart, there had been no clues before or even in the first hours after birth. Nothing they had done could have caused the defect. There was nothing they could have done to prevent it. Because of the nature of the problem, corrective surgery was impossible. Heredity did not seem to play any role at all, so future children would not face a similar danger.

The Danielses listened, asking for details and expressing their concerns. Nora wanted to know if a bad sunburn early in the pregnancy could have jeopardized the baby. Absolutely not, the doctor replied. What about her long train commute to and from work? No connection. What about the mild painkillers she'd taken for a bad headache? No relation. Paul wondered about a possible correlation with the heart attack his father had recently suffered. The doctor explained that congenital heart defects and atherosclerosis (the hardening of the arteries that typically precedes a heart attack in older persons) are entirely separate. Nora wondered if Jason had suffered. The nurse reminded her of how serene he'd been, rarely crying at all during his brief life. Paul asked whether the best thing might be another pregnancy as soon as possible. Give yourselves time, the counselor suggested.

This sort of meeting can be enormously helpful, but it can't dispel the parents' grief. Anyone who mourns for someone who has died—child, parent, spouse, or friend—goes through a sequence of emotional states. According to psychiatric research, these include: denial and isolation, anger, bargaining, depression, and acceptance.

Some parents may deny the extent of their baby's problems by insisting on more consultations, maybe a transfer to another center, perhaps a heroic operation. When they realize that nothing more can be done, they may withdraw into themselves, turning aside friends and relatives who wish to help. When they do begin to express their feelings, they often unleash intense anger, either generalized at the forces of fate or targeted at the doctors, hospital, or each other. Eventually the anger may turn inward, with self-blame festering into a lingering depression.

The physical symptoms of grief—loss of appetite, sleeplessness, fatigue, a choking sensation, shortness of breath—slowly ease. The days feel less empty as both partners return to their normal activities. But the process of grieving may last for a long time. Feelings of anger or sorrow may surface again and again, particularly on anniversaries of the baby's birth or funeral. While parents can never forget a child who died, they do eventually come to terms with their loss. "At first I couldn't think about anything but the baby," says one mother. "Then I'd think about him a couple of times an hour, then every few hours, then a few times a day, then every few days. It was like a wound, healing a little bit at a time."

• Reaching Out

It's always hard to find words of comfort after a death. When a baby dies, friends and relatives have no fond memories to recall, no words of praise and affection for the person who once was. With the best of intentions, they may make comments such as, "It was just a baby," or "There'll be other children." Such statements, meant to help, can hurt deeply, for they minimize the parents' experience and dismiss the infant as a nonperson. It's far better to communicate a simple, shared sense of sorrow and loss.

Sometimes family members of friends strip a couple's house of toys and baby furniture to make the mother's homecoming easier. Again, this well-intentioned gesture can cause more pain than solace. "When I was at the hospital, my one thought was going home where it was quiet and sitting in the beautiful little nursery we'd made. It seemed that I'd feel close to the baby there, and I'd be able to let go and mourn for her. When I got home, the nursery was bare. Everyone was trying to erase nine very meaningful months of my life."

Some women are comforted best by their own mothers and mothers-in-law, particularly if they've also lost babies. Another great source of support is parent groups sponsored by the hospital or national organizations such as HAND (Help After Neonatal Death) and AMEND (Aiding a Mother Experiencing Neonatal Death). A social worker at the medical center can put you in touch with someone who knows exactly what you're experiencing, having gone through it too.

"Usually I start by describing my own experience," explains a woman volunteer. "Then I listen. It may be the first time the mother has been able to ventilate without being afraid that someone's going to think she's crazy." Simply knowing someone who has lost a baby and slowly rebuilt her life often provides the extra hope that can make all the difference in recovering from a loss.

Friends and relatives tend to respond in ways characteristic of their personality and behavior styles. "Looking back, I could have predicted what people would say what," recalls one mother. "My parents tried to deny it ever happened. This would have been their first grandchild, and I know they didn't want me to see how disappointed they were. The friends I've always confided in were wonderful, as usual. They helped with practical things, like meals and shopping, so I could have time for myself."

Other children always feel the effects of a baby's loss, particularly if their parents don't explain what happened. A young child whose mother leaves to go to have a baby and returns distracted and sad may feel doubly abandoned—and responsible. It's not unusual for a child to have nightmares or fears that death is "catching" or that he or she will be taken to heaven just as the new baby was. If they'd resented the idea of another competitor for their parents' love, children may think that their bad thoughts killed the baby. "Death is a very scary, difficult subject for children," says a psychologist. "It's important for the parents to talk with them so they know they can talk about their little brother or sister who died. Most of all, they need to be sure that their parents still love them too."

· The Next Step

Some women, after losing a baby, are planning for the next pregnancy even before they leave the hospital. Aching with grief, they think that the sooner they get pregnant, the sooner they'll feel happy again. Yet both physiologically and psychologically, a woman needs time to recover. Obstetricians advise a wait of about a year between pregnancies. Psychologists emphasize that after any loss, the mourner needs at least six to twelve months to regain emotional equilibrium.

Even after a few months or a year, being pregnant after a loss can be emotionally wrenching. One woman compares her experience to a walk on a high and perilous tightrope. "You start off shaky, and you take one tiny step at a time. You can't relax, because you've fallen off before. You know your worst fears *can* come true. You don't trust your body, but you can't get a safety net. Once you make it past the halfway point, you may begin to feel better. But it isn't until you're safely on the other side that you can turn around and smile."

Another woman recalls how she almost danced with the joy of finding out she was pregnant the first time. The second time her reaction was quite different. "I'd lost my innocence, my naive belief in my own body. I wanted to be pregnant but I was scared the whole time. I thought, 'Oh no, here we go again.'"

Sometimes another pregnancy is neither physically nor psychologically feasible. If couples in these circumstances want a baby, adoption is often a satisfying option. By seeking out responsible persons who arrange private adoptions directly through obstetricians, they may have to wait only a few months for a baby. Adoptions through public agencies frequently take longer.

But not all couples decide to have or adopt children. "There comes a point where you have to do some soul-searching," says one woman. "I could keep getting pregnant until my uterus gave out, but I couldn't face another loss. So my husband and I talked and talked. We realized that we have a good, full life and we don't need a baby to be happy."

Such decisions are never easy. There is no right answer for all couples. If you and your partner lose a baby, you have to consider what's best for the two of you, for your other children if you have them, and for your hopes for the future. Learning as much as possible about what went wrong and why can help in making sense of the past and planning for the future. It's even more important to give yourself time to heal. Difficult as it may be, waiting will help ensure that you make a decision that's right for you and for your future children.

23 . The Next Generation: A Bright Future

Diagnosis: Destruction of red blood cells because of blood incompatibility.

Prognosis: If untreated, severe damage to the brain and other organs, which could prove fatal.

Treatment: Transfusions of fresh red blood cells.

Diagnosis: Immature lung development.

Prognosis: Risk of respiratory distress because of inability to inflate small air sacs in the lungs; potentially deadly.

Treatment: Injections of steroids to accelerate lung maturation.

Diagnosis: Heredity deficiency of an essential vitamin.

Prognosis: If uncorrected, life-threatening disruption of normal metabolism.

Treatment: Daily supplements of very high doses of the vitamin.

What is extraordinary about this list is not simply the medical problems, nor the possible outcomes, nor the available treatments, but the patients themselves. At the time of diagnosis and treatment, none of the individuals who developed these disorders, faced these risks, and underwent these therapies had yet been born.

These youngest of patients are members of the first generation of babies to be saved before their birth. In the not-distant past, they might have been doomed to lifelong impairment or death. Today they are growing up to claim a future they might never have known. Sometimes described as "miracle babies," they owe their survival not to a quirk of fate, but to decades of painstaking research in perinatology—and to recognition of the unborn as patients in their own right.

In 1971 *Williams Obstetrics*, the most widely read American textbook in the field, first articulated the new medical perspective on the fetus: "Since World War II," the editors wrote, "and especially in the last decade, knowledge of the fetus and his environment has increased remarkably. As an important consequence, the fetus has acquired status as a patient to be cared for by the physician as he long has been accustomed to caring for the mother."

In the 16th edition of *Williams,* the editors preface the text with the comment: "Happily, we have entered an era in which the fetus can be rightfully considered and treated as our second patient. . . . Fetal diagnosis and therapy have now emerged as legitimate tools the obstetrician must possess. Moreover, the number of tools the obstetrician can employ to address the needs of the fetus increases each year." They conclude that this is "the most exciting of times to be an obstetrician."

It also is the most exciting time to become a mother. If your baby, like those described at the beginning of the chapter, should develop an Rh-incompatibility problem, should face the risk of a premature birth, or should inherit a metabolic disorder, its chances of survival and long-term well-being are better than ever before. If you are diabetic, you are more likely to give birth to a normal baby than diabetic mothers of the past, largely because of new understanding of metabolism in the first weeks of gestation. The promise of having a healthy, normal baby also holds true for women with kidney problems, sickle-cell anemia, hypertension, and other chronic illnesses. And every year the promise of being "well born" is extended to thousands more. The 1980s have already brought dramatic breakthroughs in prenatal care, including pioneering operations on a fetus in order to save its life or prevent permanent damage.

Yet perinatology still has a very long way to go, both in making current treatments available to all pregnant women and in moving beyond treatment to developing effective means of prevention. The biggest problem is still preterm labor, for babies born before their time continue to face enormous risks. Since treatment after birth, even in the best of intensive-care nurseries, cannot save or protect all premature infants, prevention before birth is crucial. And, according to the experience of preterm labor centers in the U.S. and France, it also is a real possibility. At the Preterm Labor Clinic of the University of California, San Francisco, the incidence of too-early births was cut almost in half, from 6.75 percent in 1978 to 2.43 percent in 1979, after a screening, evaluation, and treatment program was set up for women at risk. A new nationwide effort to identify and educate the women most likely to begin labor early could give thousands more babies the time they need to prepare for life beyond the womb.

Medical researchers are continuing their quest for solutions to other challenging problems in perinatology, such as growth impairment before birth and infection before, during, and after delivery. But prevention of problems doesn't depend on medical advances alone. An informed woman who eats nutritiously, avoids alcohol and drugs, doesn't smoke, and gets regular prenatal checkups can do more to ensure her baby's well-being at birth than anyone else—and this holds true in most high-risk pregnancies as well as in uncomplicated ones. Of course, not all the preventable risks of pregnancy are medical. Unborn babies are extremely vulnerable to the consequences of poverty, malnutrition, and drug abuse. All too often they become the innocent victims of problems that beset not just an individual woman, but our society as a whole.

This is why the commitment to protecting children must extend beyond parents and would-be parents. "The well-being and promise of any society," the directors of the March of Dimes Birth Defects Foundation have stated, "can be measured by the health of its children." And, as perinatology has clearly demonstrated in the past decade, our children's well-being depends to a significant extent on events that occur before birth. Assuring tomorrow's children of a bright future is not just a task for perinatologists, but one for all of us. Our collective future begins with the next generation.

Appendix A • *Food Additives*

Additive	Used For	Found In
BENEFICIAL ADDITIVES		
Vitamins A and D	Fortification	Milk, margarine
Iodine	Fortification	Iodized salt
Iron, thiamin, riboflavin, niacin	Enrichment	Refined grains
Ascorbic acid (vitamin C)	Fortification, preservative	Cured meats, breakfast cereals, fruit drinks
Beta-carotene (vitamin A)	Enrichment	Margarine, butter
SAFE ADDITIVES		
Calcium propionate	Preservative	Breads, rolls, cakes, pastries
Calcium sterol lactate	Preservative	Cakes, fillings, processed egg whites, aritificial whipping cream, bread dough
EDTA	Preservative	Salad dressing, sandwich spreads, mayonnaise, canned shellfish, soft drinks
Fumaric acid	Flavoring	Powdered drinks, puddings, pie fillings
Glycerin	Preservative	Marshmallows, candy, fudge, baked goods
Lactic acid	Preservative, flavoring	Olives, frozen desserts, cheese
Gums: locust bean, arabic, furcellan, guar, acacia	Thickening	Ice cream, salad dressing, candy

Additive	Used For	Found In
LIMITED USE ONLY		
Sodium nitrite and nitrate	Preservative, color, flavoring	Hot dogs, bacon, ham, luncheon meats
MSG	Flavoring	Chinese food, processed seafood and poultry, canned foods, processed cheese, sauces
Propyl gallate	Preservative	Vegetable oils, meat products, chewing gum, chicken soup base
Sodium bisulfide, Sodium dioxide	Preservative	Dried food, wine, dehydrated potatoes
POTENTIALLY HARMFUL		
Artificial flavors and colors	Flavor and color	Candies, beverages, baked goods, gelatin desserts
Brominated vegetable oils	Stabilizer	Soft drinks
Sucrose, corn syrup, dextrose, salt	Flavoring, preservative	Processed fruit, vegetables, meats and sauces, processed desserts, candies

Appendix B . Nutrition Guides

WHEN YOU ARE PREGNANT or breast-feeding, your baby gets its food from you—most of it from what you eat meal by meal, day by day. Good nutrition is important in every pregnancy and can help minimize the risk of certain complications, such as poor fetal growth.

The following information, based on data from the University of California, San Francisco nutritionists and the California Department of Health Services, can help you eat right when you're eating for two. Use these charts daily as a guide for planning your meals. Select a variety of foods. No one food and no one food group can supply all the essential nutrients you and your baby need.

· Daily Food Guide

Food Group	Daily Servings	
	WHILE PREGNANT	WHILE BREAST-FEEDING
Protein Foods	4	4
Milk and Milk Products	4	5
Breads and Cereals	4	4
Vitamin-C-rich Fruits and Vegetables	1	1
Dark Green Vegetables	1	1
Other Fruits and Vegetables	1	1

· Protein Foods

Protein builds muscle and tissue for both you and your baby. Besides protein, *protein foods* provide B vitamins and iron. B vitamins help you obtain energy from food. Iron is needed to form red blood cells.

Protein comes from both animal and vegetable sources. Each day eat

207

a total of *4 servings*. Try to include 2 servings from animal protein foods and 2 servings from vegetable protein foods.

Animal Protein

(A serving is 2 oz. (60 g) unless otherwise noted):

Beef (ground, cube, roast, or chop)	
Clams	4 large or 9 small
Eggs	2 medium
Fish (fillet or steak)	
Fish sticks	3 sticks
Frankfurters	2
Lamb (ground, cube, roast, or chop)	
Luncheon meat	3 slices
Organ meats:	
heart, kidney, liver, tongue	
Oysters	8–12 medium
Pork, ham (ground, roast, or chop)	
Poultry:	
chicken, duck, turkey	
Rabbit	
Sausage links	4 links
Shellfish:	
crab, lobster, scallops, shrimp	
Spareribs	6 medium ribs
Tuna fish	
Veal (ground, cube, roast, or chop)	

Vegetable Protein

Beans are the best choice from vegetable protein foods. A serving of beans contains more vitamins and minerals than a serving of nuts or seeds. A serving is any of the following:

Canned beans (garbanzo, kidney, lima, pork and beans)	1 cup (240 ml)
Dried beans and peas	1 cup (240 ml)
Nut butters (cashew butter, peanut butter, etc.)	¼ cup (60 ml)
Nuts	½ cup (120 ml)
Sunflower seeds	½ cup (120 ml)
Tofu (soybean curd)	1 cup (240 ml)

You can get the protein you need by eating mainly vegetable protein foods. However, these foods should be combined with eggs and milk. Ask your doctor or dietitian/nutritionist for further information.

· Milk and Milk Products

Milk and Milk Products are the best food sources of calcium. Calcium builds strong bones and teeth in your baby. It also keeps your nerves and muscles healthy.

Milk and Milk Products also contain protein, several B vitamins, and vitamins A and D. Vitamin D helps your body use calcium. Vitamin A is needed for growth and vision. It also protects you from infection.

Choose *4 servings* of Milk and Milk Products each day if you are *pregnant*. Choose *5 servings* if you are *breast-feeding*. A serving is 1 cup (8 oz. or 240 ml) unless otherwise noted.

Cheese (except Camembert, cream)	1 slice (1½ oz. or 45 g)
Cheese spread	4 tablespoons (60 ml)
Cocoa made with milk	1¼ cups (10 oz. or 300 ml)
Cottage cheese	1⅓ cups (320 ml)
Custard (flan)	
Ice cream	1½ cups (360 ml)
Ice milk	
Milk	
buttermilk	
chocolate (not drink)	1¼ cups (10 oz. or 300 ml)
evaporated	½ cup (4 oz. or 120 ml)
goat	
low-fat	
non-fat	
non-fat (made from dry milk powder)	
non-fat dry milk powder	⅓ cup (80 ml)
whole	
Milkshake	
Pudding	
Soups made with milk	1½ cups (12 oz. or 360 ml)
Yogurt (plain)	

Not all Milk and Milk Products contain vitamins A and D. Check the label!

· Breads and Cereals

Breads and Cereals have several nutrients important for you and your baby including B vitamins and iron. These foods may be either whole grain or enriched. It's best to eat whole grains—they contain more vitamins and minerals. Whole grains also provide fiber, which helps prevent constipation.

Choose *4 servings* of Breads and Cereals each day. A serving is any of the following:

Whole Grain Items

Bread: cracked, whole wheat, or rye	1 slice
Cereal, hot: oatmeal (rolled oats), rolled wheat, cracked wheat, wheat and malted barley	½ cup cooked (120 ml)
Cereal, ready-to-eat: puffed oats, shredded wheat, wheat flakes, granola	¾ cup (180 ml)
Rice (brown)	½ cup cooked (120 ml)
Wheat germ	1 tablespoon (15 ml)

In some communities you can also buy whole wheat macaroni, noodles, spaghetti, and tortillas.

Enriched Items

Bagel	1 small
Bread (all except those listed above)	1 slice
Cereal, hot: cream of wheat, cream of rice, farina, cornmeal, grits	½ cup cooked (120 ml)
Cereal, ready-to-eat (all except those listed above)	¾ cup (180 ml)
Crackers	4
Macaroni, noodles, spaghetti	½ cup cooked (120 ml)
Pancake, waffle	1 medium (5-inch or 13-cm diameter)
Rice (white)	½ cup cooked
Roll, biscuit, muffin, dumpling	1
Tortilla	1 (6-inch or 15-cm diameter)

Doughnuts, cakes, pies, and cookies are not included in the Breads and Cereals group. These foods contain mostly calories and very few nutrients.

· Fruits and Vegetables (Listed by nutrient content)

Vitamin-C-Rich Fruits and Vegetables contain ascorbic acid (vitamin C). This vitamin is needed to hold body cells together and to strengthen blood vessel walls. Ascorbic acid also aids in healing wounds.

Choose *2 servings* of Vitamin-C-Rich Fruits and Vegetables each day. A serving is ¾ cup (180 ml) unless otherwise noted.

Vegetables

Bok choy	
Broccoli	1 stalk
Brussels sprouts	3–4
Cabbage	
Cauliflower	
Chili peppers (green or red)	¼ cup
Greens: collard, kale, mustard, turnip	
Peppers (green or red)	½ medium
Tomatoes	2 medium
Watercress	

Fruits

Cantaloupe	½ medium
Grapefruit	½ large
Guava	½ small
Mango	1 medium
Orange	1 medium
Papaya	½ small
Strawberries	
Tangerine	2 large

Juices

Fruit juices and drinks with vitamin C added	
Grapefruit	½ cup (4 oz. or 120 ml)
Orange	½ cup (4 oz. or 120 ml)
Pineapple	1½ cups (12 oz. or 360 ml)
Tomato	1½ cups (12 oz. or 360 ml)

Dark Green Vegetables are an excellent source of vitamin A and folacin. Your baby needs vitamin A for bone growth and tooth formation. Vitamin A is also important for vision and resisting infections.

Folacin, a B vitamin, is needed to form red blood cells and other body cells. Cooking temperatures destroy folacin, so eat Dark Green Vegetables raw whenever possible.

Choose *1 serving* of Dark Green Vegetables each day. A serving is 1 cup (240 ml) raw or ¾ cup (180 ml) cooked.

Asparagus	Greens: beet, collard,
Bok choy	kale, mustard, turnip
Broccoli	Lettuce (dark leafy:
Brussels sprouts	red leaf, romaine)
Cabbage	Scallions
Chicory	Spinach
Endive	Swiss chard
Escarole	Watercress

Other Fruits and Vegetables add vitamins and minerals to your diet. Those dark yellow in color contain vitamin A. Fruits and vegetables also provide fiber, which is important for normal bowel movements.

Choose *1 serving* of Other Fruits and Vegetables each day. A serving is ½ cup (120 ml) unless otherwise noted.

Vegetables

Artichoke	1 medium
Bamboo shoots	
Beans (green, wax)	
Bean sprouts	
Beet	
Burdock root	
Carrot	
Cauliflower	
Celery	
Corn	
Cucumber	
Eggplant	
Hominy	
Lettuce (head, Boston, Bibb)	
Mushrooms	
Nori seaweed	
Onion	
Parsnip	
Peas	
Pea pods	
Potato	1 medium
Radishes	
Summer squash	
Sweet potato	1 medium
Winter squash	
Yam	1 medium
Zucchini	

Fruits

Apple	1 medium
Apricot	2 medium
Banana	1 small
Berries	
Cherries	
Dates	5
Figs	2 large
Fruit cocktail	
Grapes	
Kumquats	3
Nectarine	2 medium
Peach	1 medium
Pear	1 medium
Persimmon	1 small
Pineapple	
Plums	2 medium
Prunes	4 medium
Pumpkin	¼ cup (60 ml)
Raisins	
Watermelon	

Dark yellow fruits and vegetables are an excellent source of vitamin A. These include carrots, sweet potatoes, yams, winter squash, apricots, persimmons, and pumpkin.

• Sample Meals

The following suggestions may help you in your meal planning while pregnant and while breast-feeding:

	Pregnant Woman	Nursing Woman
BREAKFAST:	1 svg. vitamin-C-rich fruits and vegetables 1 svg. grain products 1 svg. milk and milk products	1 svg. vitamin-C-rich fruits and vegetables 1 svg. grain products 1 svg. milk and milk products
MORNING SNACK:	Optional (fruit)	Optional (fruit)
LUNCH:	2 svgs. grain products 1 svg. protein foods 1 svg. other fruits and vegetables 1 svg. milk and milk products	2 svgs. grain products 1 svg. protein foods 1 svg. other fruits and vegetables 1 svg. milk and milk products

	Pregnant Woman	**Nursing Woman**
AFTERNOON SNACK:	1 svg. protein foods ½ svg. milk and milk products	1 svg. protein foods 1 svg. milk and milk products
DINNER:	2 svgs. protein foods 2 svgs. leafy green vegetables 1 svg. milk and milk products	2 svgs. protein foods 2 svgs. leafy green vegetables 1 svg. milk and milk products
EVENING SNACK:	½ svg. milk and milk products	1 svg. milk and milk products
BREAKFAST:	4 oz. orange juice ½ cup oatmeal with brown sugar 8 oz. milk coffee or tea	4 oz. orange juice ½ cup oatmeal with brown sugar 8 oz. milk coffee or tea
MORNING SNACK:	Optional (fruit)	Optional (fruit)
LUNCH:	1 tuna fish sandwich made with: 2 slices whole wheat bread ½ cup tuna fish diced celery and onion to taste, mayonnaise, lettuce 1 small banana 8 oz. milk	1 tuna fish sandwich made with: 2 slices whole wheat bread ½ cup tuna fish diced celery and onion to taste, mayonnaise, lettuce 1 small banana 8 oz. milk
AFTERNOON SNACK:	½ cup salted peanuts 4 oz. milk	½ cup salted peanuts 8 oz. milk
DINNER:	6 oz. roast beef ½ cup egg noodles with sautéed poppy seeds ¾ cup cut asparagus salad made with: 1 cup torn spinach sliced mushrooms and radishes to taste oil and vinegar 8 oz. milk coffee or tea	6 oz. roast beef ½ cup egg noodles with sautéed poppy seeds ¾ cup cut asparagus salad made with: 1 cup torn spinach sliced mushrooms and radishes to taste oil and vinegar 8 oz. milk coffee or tea
EVENING SNACK:	2 oatmeal raisin cookies 4 oz. milk	2 oatmeal raisin cookies 8 oz. milk

Appendix C . A Perinatal Glossary

abortion. The termination, spontaneous or induced, of pregnancy at any time before the fetus has attained a stage of viability, i.e., before it is capable of extrauterine existence.

abruptio placentae. Premature separation of normally implanted placenta.

alpha fetal protein (AFP). A protein manufactured mainly in the liver of a fetus and released into the amniotic fluid when the fetus urinates.

amniocentesis. Prenatal diagnostic test; sampling of the amniotic fluid that surrounds a fetus in order to obtain information about its well-being.

amniotic sac. The "bag of waters" containing the fetus before delivery.

amniotomy. Artificial rupture of the membranes to induce labor.

analgesic. Drug which relieves pain, used during labor.

anencephaly. Form of anomaly with absence of a brain.

anomaly. Malformation.

anoxia. Oxygen deficiency; any condition of absence of tissue oxidation.

antenatal. Occurring or formed before birth.

antepartal. Before labor and delivery or childbirth; prenatal.

antibody. A protein manufactured by the body's protective immune system that reacts specifically against the foreign substance that initially triggered its production.

asphyxia. Anoxia and carbon dioxide retention resulting from failure of respiration.

bag of waters. The membranes which enclose the amniotic fluid.

Braxton Hicks. Painless uterine contractions occurring periodically throughout pregnancy.

breech delivery. Labor and delivery marked by breech presentations (buttocks or feet first).

cephalic. Belonging to the head.

cephalic presentation. Presentation of any part of the fetal head in labor.

cephalo-pelvic disproportion. A complication of labor in which the baby's head is too large to pass through the birth canal.

cerclage. A suture placed around an "incompetent" cervix to prevent a miscarriage.

cervix. A necklike part; the lower and narrow end of the uterus.

cesarean. Surgical delivery of a baby through the uterus and abdomen.

chromosome. One of several small, dark-staining and more or less rod-shaped bodies which appear in the nucleus of the cell at the time of cell division.

colostrum. A substance in the first milk after delivery, giving it a yellowish color.

conception. The impregnation of the female ovum by the sperm of the male, resulting in a new being.

condyloma. (*pl.* condylomata) A wartlike growth near the anus or the vulva.

congenital. Born with the person; existing from or before birth, as, for example, congenital disease originating in the fetus before birth.

corpus luteum. The yellow mass found in the ovary after the ovum has been expelled.

delivery. The expulsion of a child by the mother or its extraction by the obstetric practitioner. The removal of a part from the body; as *delivery* of the placenta.

dizygotic. Pertaining to or proceeding from two zygotes (two eggs or ova).

eclampsia. Once called acute "toxemia of pregnancy"; characterized by convulsions and coma which may occur during pregnancy or labor.

ectopic. Out of place.

ectopic pregnancy. Gestation in which the fetus is out of its normal place in the cavity of the uterus. It includes gestation in the fallopian tube or in a rudimentary horn of the uterus (cornual pregnancy); cervical pregnancy; and abdominal and ovarian pregnancy.

effacement. Obliteration. In obstetrics, refers to thinning and shortening of the cervix.

ejaculation. A sudden act of expulsion, as of semen.

electronic fetal monitoring. A method of checking a baby's well-being before or during labor by checking its heart rate and response to contractions.

embryo. The product of conception in utero from the third through the fifth week of gestation; after that length of time, it is called the fetus.

endometrium. The mucous membrane which lines the uterus.

engagement. In obstetrics, applies to the entrance of the presenting part into the superior pelvic strait and the beginning of the descent through the pelvic canal.

episiotomy. Surgical incision of the vaginal orifice for delivery of a baby.

erythroblastosis fetalis. A severe disease of the newborn, due to Rh incompatibility.

estriol. The form of estrogen that increases most dramatically in pregnancy.

fertility. The ability to produce offspring; power of reproduction.

fertilization. The fusion of the sperm with the ovum; it marks the beginning of pregnancy.

fetoscopy. A prenatal diagnostic test in which physicians use sophisticated, still-experimental techniques to peer into the womb.

fetus. The baby in utero from the end of the fifth week of gestation until birth.

forceps. Metal devices used to protect a baby's head and guide it through the lower birth canal.

fundus. The upper rounded portion of the uterus between the points of insertion of the fallopian tubes.

gamete. A sexual cell; an unfertilized egg or a mature sperm cell.

gene. A hereditary factor in the chromosome which carries on a hereditary, transmissible character.

gonad. A gamete-producing gland; an ovary or testis.

hormone. A chemical substance produced in an organ, which, when carried to an associated organ by the blood stream, stimulates a functional activity.

human chorionic gonadotropin (HCG). Characteristic hormone of early pregnancy.

human placental lactogen (HPL). A protein produced only in pregnancy. HPL levels in the mother's blood generally increase until the 37th week and then level off.

hydatidiform mole. Cystic proliferation of chorionic villi resembling a bunch of grapes, arising from placental tissue.

hydramnios. An excessive amount of amniotic fluid.

hydrocephalus. Excessive fluid within the skull.

hypoxia. Insufficient oxygen to support normal metabolic requirements.

intrauterine transfusion. Injection of blood cells into a fetus, usually performed for babies with Rh incompatibility.

ketoacidosis. A build-up of weak acids called ketones when the body is deprived of glucose and begins to break down stored fat for energy use.

labor. The series of processes by which the products of conception are expelled from the mother's body.

lactation. The act or period of giving milk; the secretion of milk; the time or period of secreting milk.

lanugo. The fine hair on the body of the fetus.

lecithin/sphingomyelin ratio. A test of fetal lung maturity by measuring the amounts of lecithin, a fat produced by the lungs, and sphingomyelin, a fat produced by the skin.

linea nigra. A dark line appearing on the abdomen and extending from the pubis toward the umbilicus, considered one of the signs of pregnancy.

lochia. The discharge from the genital canal during several days subsequent to delivery.

meconium. The dark-green or black substance found in the large intestine of the fetus or newly born infant.

menarche. The establishment or the beginning of the menstrual function.

menopause. The period at which menstruation ceases; the "change of life."

miscarriage. Death of a fetus prior to the twentieth week of gestation; spontaneous abortion.

molding. The shaping of the baby's head so as to adjust itself to the size and shape of the birth canal.

monozygotic. Pertaining to or derived from one zygote, or one egg or ovum.

multigravida. A woman who has been pregnant several times or many times.

multipara. A woman who has borne several children.

neonatal. Pertaining to the newborn, usually for the first four weeks of life.

neonatology. Subspecialty of pediatrics dedicated to caring for sick babies in their first days of life.

nonstress testing (NST). A method of assessing fetal well-being by monitoring its heart rate and response to spontaneous movements or contractions.

nullipara. A woman who has not borne children.

ovary. The sexual gland of the female in which the ova are developed. There are two ovaries, one at each side of the pelvis.

ovulation. The release of an ovum from the ovary.

ovum. The female reproductive cell. The human ovum is a round cell about 1/120 of an inch in diameter, developed in the ovary.

oxytocin. One of the two hormones secreted by the posterior pituitary; it induces contractions of the uterus.

parity. The condition of a woman with respect to her having borne children.

perinatal. Before, during and immediately after birth.

perinatology. Subspecialty of obstetrics dedicated to care of high-risk mothers and their unborn babies; also called maternal-fetal medicine.

perineum. The area between the vagina and the rectum.

Pitocin. A synthetic solution of oxytocin.

placenta. The circular flat, vascular structure in the impregnated uterus forming the principal medium of communication between the mother and the fetus.

placenta previa. A placenta which is implanted in the lower uterine segment so that it adjoins or covers the cervix.

placental abruption. Premature separation of the normally implanted placenta.

postmaturity. A condition that occurs in some pregnancies that continue beyond the forty-week term, when the placenta can no longer supply adequate nutrients to the fetus.

postnatal. Occurring after birth.

postpartal. After delivery or childbirth.

presentation. Term used to designate the position of the fetus as felt by the physician's examining finger when introduced into the cervix.

preterm labor. Onset of rhythmic contractions after the twentieth and before the thirty-seventh week of pregnancy.

primigravida A woman who is pregnant for the first time.

progesterone. The pure hormone whose function is to prepare the endometrium for the reception and development of the fertilized ovum; it also helps to maintain the pregnancy.

proteinuria. High levels of protein in urine.

puerperium. The period elapsing between the termination of labor and the return of the uterus to its normal condition, about six weeks.

quickening. The mother's first perception of the movements of the fetus.

Rh. Abbreviation for Rhesus, a type of monkey. This term is used for a property of human blood cells, because of its relationship to a similar property in the blood cells of Rhesus monkeys.

RhoGAM. A substance containing anti-RH antibodies given to Rh-negative women after delivery, abortion, or miscarriage to prevent the production of these antibodies, which could threaten any Rh-positive babies these women might conceive in the future.

rubella. German measles.

scalp sampling. A test of a baby's condition during labor by obtaining a sample of blood from a blood vessel on its scalp. The physician uses an amnioscope (a cone-shaped device with an attached light source) to view the baby and a scalpel to prick its blood vessel.

small-for-gestational age (SGA). A baby who weighs less than do 90 percent of babies at the same stage of pregnancy or at delivery.

stillborn. Born without life.

stress testing. A method of assessing fetal well-being by monitoring fetal heart rate and its response to contractions induced by oxytocin.

teratogen. Any substance that causes deformities in an unborn baby.

ultrasound (sonography). High-frequency sound waves used to evaluate fetal well-being and diagnose structural defects.

uterus. The hollow muscular organ in the female designed for the lodgment and nourishment of the fetus during its development until birth.

vagina. The canal in the female extending from the vulva to the cervix of the uterus.

version. The act of turning; specifically, a turning of the fetus in the uterus so as to change the presenting part and bring it into more favorable position for delivery.

vertex. In anatomy, the top or crown of the head.

viable. A term in medical jurisprudence signifying "able or likely to live"; applied to the condition of the child at birth.

zygote. A cell resulting from the fusion of two gametes.

Appendix D • Perinatal and Neonatal Centers in the United States

This listing is reprinted with permission from Ross Planning Associates of Ross Laboratories, Columbus, Ohio.

ALABAMA

Brookwood Medical Center
2010 Brookwood Medical Center Dr.
Birmingham, AL 35209
205-877-1000

Children's Hospital
1601 Sixth Ave. S.
Birmingham, AL 35233
205-933-4000

Cooper Green Hospital
1515 Sixth Ave. S.
Birmingham, AL 35233
205-933-9211

University of Alabama Hospital
University Station
521 S. Nineteenth St.
Birmingham, AL 35294
205-934-4011

Huntsville Hospital
101 Sivley Rd.
Huntsville, AL 35801
205-533-8020

University of Southern Alabama
2451 Fillingim St.
Mobile, AL 36617
205-471-7000

Baptist Medical Center
2105 E. South Blvd.
Montgomery, AL 36198
205-288-2100

St. Margaret's Hospital
834 Adams Ave.
Box 311
Montgomery, AL 36104
205-269-8000

Druid City Hospital Regional Medical Center
809 University Blvd. E.
Tuscaloosa, AL 35401
205-759-7111

ALASKA

Providence Hospital
3200 Providence Dr.
Anchorage, AK 99504
907-276-4511

ARIZONA

Flagstaff Hospital and Medical Center of Northern Arizona
1215 N. Beaver St.
Box 1268
Flagstaff, AZ 86002
602-744-5233

Desert Samaritan Hospital
1400 S. Dobson Rd.
Mesa, AZ 85202
602-835-3000

Good Samaritan Hospital
1033 McDowell Rd.
Phoenix, AZ 85006
602-257-2000

John C. Lincoln Hospital
9211 N. Second St.
Phoenix, AZ 85020
602-934-2381

Maricopa County General Hospital
2601 E. Roosevelt St.
Phoenix, AZ 85008
602-267-5411

St. Joseph Hospital and Medical Center
Box 2071
Phoenix, AZ 85001
602-241-3000

Scottsdale Memorial Hospital
7400 E. Osborn Rd.
Scottsdale, AZ 85251
602-994-9616

Arizona Health Sciences Center
1501 N. Campbell
Tucson, AZ 85724
602-626-6000

Tucson Medical Center
E. Grant and Beverly Rds.
Tucson, AZ 85733
602-327-5461

ARKANSAS

Union Medical Center
700 W. Grove St.
El Dorado, AR 71730
501-864-3200

Washington Regional Medical Center
1125 N. College Ave.
Fayetteville, AR 72701
501-442-1000

St. Edward Mercy Medical Center
7301 Rogers Ave.
Fort Smith, AR 72903
501-452-5100

Arkansas Children's Hospital
804 Wolfe St.
Little Rock, AR 72201
501-370-1100

Baptist Medical Center
9601 Interstate 630
Little Rock, AR 72201
501-227-2200

Doctors Hospital
W. Capitol at University Ave.
Little Rock, AR 72205
501-661-4000

St. Vincent's Infirmary
Markham and University Ave.
Little Rock, AR 72201
501-661-3000

University of Arkansas Medical Center
4301 W. Markham St.
Little Rock, AR 72201
501-661-5000

CALIFORNIA

Kern Medical Center
1830 Flower St.
Bakersfield, CA 93305
805-326-2000

Kaiser Foundation Hospital
9400 E. Rosecrans Ave.
Bellflower, CA 90706
213-920-4811

Alta Bates Hospital
3001 Colby St. at Ashby
Berkeley, CA 94705
415-845-7110

El Centro Community Hospital
1415 Ross Avenue
El Centro, CA 92243
714-352-7111

Kaiser Foundation Hospital
9961 Sierra Ave.
Fontana, CA
714-829-5000

Valley Children's Hospital
3151 N. Milbrook Ave.
Fresno, CA 93703
209-225-3000

Valley Medical Center of Fresno
445 S. Cedar Ave.
Fresno, CA 93702
209-453-4000

Glendale Adventist Medical Center
1509 Wilson Terrace
Glendale, CA 91206
213-240-8000

Centinela Hospital Medical Center
555 E. Hardy
Inglewood, CA 90301
213-673-4660

Daniel Freeman Memorial Hospital
333 N. Prairie Ave.
Box 100
Inglewood, CA 90306
213-674-7050

Loma Linda University Medical Center
  Women's Hospital
  Miller Children's Hospital
11234 Anderson St.
Loma Linda, CA 92350
714-796-7311

Memorial Hospital Medical Center of Long Beach
2801 Atlantic Ave.
Long Beach, CA 90801
213-595-2311

Cedars-Sinai Medical Center
8700 Beverly Blvd.
Los Angeles, CA 90048
213-855-5000

Children's Hospital of Los Angeles
4650 Sunset Blvd.
Los Angeles, CA 90027
213-660-2450

Hollywood Presbyterian Medical Center
1300 N. Vermont Ave.
Los Angeles, CA 90027
213-660-3530

Kaiser Foundation Hospital
4867 Sunset Blvd.
Los Angeles, CA 90027
213-667-8101

Los Angeles County–
University of Southern
California Medical Center
(Women's Hospital)
1240 Mission Rd.
Los Angeles, CA 90033
213-226-3427

Martin Luther King General
Hospital
12021 S. Wilmington Ave.
Los Angeles, CA 90059
213-603-5201

University of California at
Los Angeles Medical School
10833 LeConte Ave.
Los Angeles, CA 90024
213-825-6301

White Memorial Medical
Center
1720 Brooklyn Ave.
Los Angeles, CA 90033
213-268-5000

St. Francis Medical Center
3630 E. Imperial Hwy.
Lynwood, CA 90262
213-603-6000

Contra Costa Medical
Services
2500 Alhambra Ave.
Martinez, CA 94553
415-372-4261

Modesto City Hospital
730 Seventeenth St.
Modesto, CA 95354
209-577-2100

Children's Hospital Medical
Center of Northern California
Fifty-first and Grove Sts.
Oakland, CA 94609
415-428-3000

Kaiser Foundation Hospital
280 W. McArthur Blvd.
Oakland, CA 94611
415-428-5000

Naval Regional Medical
Center
8750 Mountain Blvd.
Oakland, CA 94627
415-639-2357

Children's Hospital of Orange
County
1109 W. LaVeta Ave.
Orange, CA 92668
714-997-3000

University of California
Irvine Medical Center
101 City Dr. S.
Orange, CA 92668
714-634-6011

Kaiser Foundation Hospital
13652 Cantara St.
Panorama City, CA 91402
213-908-2000

Huntington Memorial
Hospital
100 Congress St.
Pasadena, CA 91105
213-440-5000

Pomona Valley Community
Hospital
1798 N. Garey Ave.
Box 2766
Pomona, CA 91766
714-623-8715

Mercy Medical Center
Clairmont Heights
Redding, CA 96001
916-243-2121

Riverside General Hospital–
University Medical Center
9851 Magnolia Ave.
Riverside, CA 92503
714-351-7100

The Perinatal Center
Sutter Community Hospital
Fifty-second and F St.
Sacramento, CA 95819
916-454-3450

University of California
Davis Medical Center
2315 Stockton Blvd.
Sacramento, CA 95817
916-453-2011

San Bernardino County
Medical Center
780 E. Gilbert St.
San Bernardino, CA 92404
714-383-3115

Children's Hospital
8001 Frost St.
San Diego, CA 92123
714-292-3111

Mercy Hospital and Medical
Center
4077 Fifth Ave.
San Diego, CA 92103
714-294-8111

Naval Regional Medical
Center
San Diego, CA 92134
714-233-2411

University Hospital
University of California
Medical Center
225 W. Dickinson St.
San Diego, CA 92103
714-294-6222

Children's Hospital of San
Francisco
3700 California St.
San Francisco, CA 94119
415-387-8700

Kaiser Foundation Hospital
2425 Geary Blvd.
San Francisco, CA 94115
415-929-4000

Letterman Army Medical
Center
The Presidio
San Francisco, CA 94129
415-561-2830

Mt. Zion Hospital and
Medical Center
1600 Divisadero St.
San Francisco, CA 94120
415-567-6600

St. Luke's Hospital
3555 Army St.
San Francisco, CA 94110
415-647-6800

San Francisco General
Hospital Medical Center
1001 Potrero Ave.
San Francisco, CA 94110
415-821-8200

University of California
Medical Center
H. C. Moffit Hospital
Third and Parnassus Ave.
San Francisco, CA 94143
415-666-1401

Alexian Brothers Hospital
225 N. Jackson Ave.
San Jose, CA 95116
408-259-5000

Good Samaritan Hospital of Santa Clara Valley
2425 Samaritan Dr.
San Jose, CA 95124
408-559-2011

Santa Clara Valley Medical Center
751 S. Bascom Ave.
San Jose, CA 95128
408-279-5100

Santa Teresa Community Hospital
250 Hospital Pkwy.
San Jose, CA 95123
408-578-4444

Marin General Hospital
250 Bon Air Rd.
San Rafael, CA 94901
415-461-0100

Kaiser Permanente Medical Center
900 Kiely Blvd.
Santa Clara, CA 95051
408-985-4000

Community Hospital
3325 Chanate Rd.
Santa Rosa, CA 95404
707-544-3340

Stanford University Medical Center
Stanford, CA 93405
415-497-2300

Medical Center of Tarzana
18321 Clark St.
Tarzana, CA 91356
213-881-0800

Harbor General Hospital
1000 W. Carson St.
Torrance, CA 90509
213-533-2345

Little Company of Mary Hospital
4101 Torrance Blvd.
Torrance, CA 90503
213-540-7676

David Grant USAF Medical Center
Travis Air Force Base, CA 94535
707-438-2625

Kaiser Foundation Hospital
13652 Cantara St.
Van Nuys, CA 91402
213-908-2822

General Hospital, Ventura County
3291 Loma Vsita Rd.
Ventura, CA 93003
805-648-6181

Kaweah Delta District Hospital
400 W. Mineral King St.
Visalia, CA 93291
209-625-2211

Queen of the Valley Hospital
1115 S. Sunset Ave.
Box 1980
West Covina, CA 91793
213-962-4011

Presbyterian Intercommunity Hospital
12401 E. Washington Blvd.
Whittier, CA 90602
213-698-0811

COLORADO

Fitzsimons Army Medical Center
Aurora, CO 80045
303-341-8035

Memorial Hospital
1400 E. Boulder St.
Box 1326
Colorado Springs, CO 80901
303-475-5011

Children's Hospital Presbyterian St. Luke's Medical Center
1056 E. Nineteenth Ave.
Denver, CO 80218
303-861-8888

Denver General Hospital
W. Eighth Ave. and Cherokee
Denver, CO 80204
303-893-6000

Rose Medical Center
4567 E. Ninth Ave.
Denver, CO 80220
303-320-2121

St. Joseph Hospital
1835 Franklin St.
Denver, CO 80218
303-837-7111

University of Colorado Health Sciences Center
4200 E. Ninth Ave.
Denver, CO 80262
303-399-1222

La Plata Community Hospital
3801 N. Main Ave.
Durango, CO 81301
303-259-1110

Poudre Valley Hospital
1024 Lemay Ave.
Fort Collins, CO 80524
303-482-4111

St. Mary's Hospital and Medical Center
Seventh St. and Patterson Rd.
Box 1628
Grand Junction, CO 81502
303-244-2273

Weld County General Hospital
Sixteenth St. and Seventeenth Ave.
Greeley, CO 80631
303-352-4121

St. Mary-Corwin Hospital
1008 Minnequa Ave.
Pueblo, CO 81004
303-560-4000

Lutheran Medical Center
8300 W. Thirty-eighth Ave.
Wheatridge, CO 80033
303-425-4500

CONNECTICUT

Bridgeport Hospital
267 Grant St.
Bridgeport, CT 06610
203-384-3000

Danbury Hospital
24 Hospital Ave.
Danbury, CT 06810
203-797-7000

University of Connecticut Health Center
John Dempsey Hospital
Farmington, CT 06032
203-674-2000

Hartford Hospital
80 Seymour St.
Hartford, CT 06115
203-524-3011

Mount Sinai Hospital
500 Blue Hills Ave.
Hartford, CT 06112
203-242-4431

St. Francis Hospital and
Medical Center
114 Woodland St.
Hartford, CT 06105
203-548-4000

Yale–New Haven Hospital
789 Howard Ave.
New Haven, CT 06504
203-785-4242

DELAWARE

Wilmington Medical Center
501 W. Fourteenth St.
Box 1668
Wilmington, DE 19899
302-428-1212

DISTRICT OF COLUMBIA

Children's Hospital National
Medical Center
111 Michigan Ave. NW
Washignton, DC 20010
202-745-5000

Columbia Hospital for
Women
2425 L St. NW
Washington, DC 20037
202-293-6500

George Washington
University Hospital
901 Twenty-third St. NW
Washington, DC 20037
202-676-5000

Georgetown University
Hospital
3800 Reservoir Rd. NW
Washington, DC 20007
202-625-7745

Howard University Hospital
2041 Georgia Ave. NW
Washington, DC 20060
202-745-1595

Walter Reed Army Medical
Center
Washington, DC 20012
202-576-1057

FLORIDA

Halifax Hospital Medical
Center
Clyde Morris Blvd.
Box 1990
Daytona Beach, FL 32015

Broward General Medical
Center
1600 S. Andrews Ave.
Fort Lauderdale, FL 33316
305-463-3131

University of Florida College
of Medicine
Shands Teaching Hospital
Box J-296 JHMHC
Gainesville, FL 32610
904-392-3701

Baptist Medical Center
800 Prudential Dr.
Jacksonville, FL 32207
315-463-3131

University Hospital of
Jacksonville
655 Eighth St. W.
Jacksonville, FL 32209
904-358-3272

Lakeland General Hospital
Lakeland Hills Blvd.
Drawer 448
Lakeland, FL 33802
813-683-0411

Baptist Hospital of Miami
8900 N. Kendall Dr.
Miami, FL 33176
305-596-1960

University of Miami
Jackson Memorial Hospital
Medical Center
1611 NW Twelfth Ave.
Miami, FL 33136
305-325-7429

Variety Children's Hospital
6125 SW Thirty-first St.
Miami, FL 33155
305-666-6511

Florida Hospital/Orlando
601 E. Rollins Ave.
Orlando, FL 32803
305-896-6611

Orlando Regional Medical
Center
1414 Kuhl Ave.
Orlando, FL 32806
305-841-5111

Sacred Heart Hospital
5151 N. Ninth Ave.
Pensacola, FL 32503
904-476-7851

All Children's Hospital
801 Sixth St.
St. Petersburg, FL 33701
813-898-7451

Bayfront Medical Center
701 Sixth St. S.
St. Petersburg, FL 33701
813-823-1234

Tampa General Hospital
Davis Islands
Tampa, FL 33606
813-253-0711

GEORGIA

Phoebe Putney Memorial
Hospital
417 Third Ave.
Box 1828
Albany, GA 31703
912-883-1800

Americus and Sumter County
Hospital
712 Forsythe St.
Americus, GA 31709
912-924-6011

Athens General Hospital
797 Cobb St.
Athens, GA 30606
404-549-9977

St. Mary's Hospital of Athens,
Inc.
1230 Baxter St.
Athens, GA 30613
404-548-7581

Crawford W. Long Memorial
Hospital of Emory University
35 Linden Ave. NE
Atlanta, GA 30365
404-892-4411

Georgia Baptist Hospital
300 Blvd. NE
Atlanta, Ga 30312
404-653-4200

Grady Memorial Hospital
80 Butler St. SE
Atlanta, GA 30335
404-588-4307

Henrietta Egleston Hospital
for Children, Inc.
1405 Clifton Rd. NE
Atlanta, GA 30322
404-325-6000

Hughes Spalding Pavilion
35 Butler St. SE
Atlanta, GA 30335
404-659-8181

Northside Hospital
1000 Johnson Ferry Rd. NE
Atlanta, GA 30042
404-256-8000

Piedmont Hospital
1968 Peachtree Rd. NW
Atlanta, GA 30309
404-355-7611

Southwest Community
Hospital
501 Fairborn Rd. SW
Atlanta, GA 30331
404-344-7110

Medical College of Georgia
Eugene Talmadge Memorial
Hospital and Clinics
1120 Fifteenth St.
Augusta, GA 30912
404-828-0211 (Hospital)
414-828-3466 (Medical
College)

University Hospital
1350 Walton Way
Augusta, GA 30910
404-722-9011

Cobb General Hospital
3950 Austell Rd.
Austell, GA 30001
404-941-0400

Glynn-Brunswick Memorial
Hospital
2515 Parkwood Dr.
Box 1518
Brunswick, GA 31520
912-264-6960

Tanner Memorial Hospital
705 Dixie St.
Carrollton, GA 30117
404-834-8811

The Medical Center of
Columbus, Georgia
710 Center St.
Columbus, GA 31994
404-324-4711

Hamilton Memorial Hospital
Memorial Drive
P.O. Box 1168
Dalton, GA 30720
404-278-2105

DeKalb General Hospital
2701 N. Decatur Rd.
Decatur, GA 30033
404-292-4444

Joan Glancy Memorial
Hospital
W. Lawrenceville Hwy.
Duluth, GA 30136
404-476-3751

John L. Hutchinson Memorial
Tri-County Hospital
100 Gross Crescent
Fort Oglethorpe, GA 30742
404-866-2121

Northeast Georgia Medical
Center
743 Spring St. NE
Gainesville, GA 30505
404-535-3553

Griffin-Spalding County Hospital
S. Eighth St.
Griffin, GA 30223
404-228-2721

West Georgia Medical Center
1514 Vernon Rd.
Box 1567
La Grange, GA 30240
404-882-1411

Medical Center of Central Georgia
777 Hemlock St.
Macon, GA 31208
912-744-1000

Kennestone Hospital
677 Church St.
Marietta, GA 30060
404-424-8522

Cowetta General Hospital
Hospital Rd.
Box 2228
Newnan, GA 30264
404-253-1912

Clayton General Hospital
11 SW Upper Riverdale Rd.
Box 328
Riverdale, GA 30274
404-478-1770

Floyd Medical Center
Turner McCall Blvd.
Box 233
Rome, GA 30161
404-295-5500

Candler General Hospital
601 Abercorn St.
Box 9787
Savannah, GA 31412
912-354-9211

Memorial Medical Center
P.O. Box 23089
Savannah, GA 31403
912-356-8000

Upson County Hospital
801 W. Gordon St.
Box 1059
Thomaston, GA 30286
404-647-8111

John D. Archbold Memorial Hospital
Gordon Ave. and Mimosa Dr.
Box 1018
Thomasville, GA 31792
912-226-4121

Tift General Hospital
901 E. Eighteenth St.
Drawer 747
Tifton, GA 31793
912-382-7120

Stephens County Hospital
Falls Rd.
Box 947
Toccoa, GA 30577
404-886-6841

South Georgia Medical Center
Pendleton Park
Box 1727
Valdosta, GA 31601
912-242-3450

Houston County Hospital Complex
1601 Watson Blvd.
Box 2886
Warner Robins, GA 31093
912-922-4281

Memorial Hospital
410 Darling Ave.
Box 139
Waycross, GA 31501
912-283-3030

HAWAII

Kapiolani Children's Medical
Center
1319 Punahou St.
Honolulu, HI 96525
808-947-8511

Tripler Army Medical Center
Honolulu, HI 96859
808-433-6661

IDAHO

St. Luke's Regional Medical
Center
190 E. Bannock St.
Boise, ID 83702
208-386-2222

St. Joseph's Hospital, Inc.
415 Sixth St.
Lewiston, ID 83501
208-743-2511

Bannock Memorial Hospital
Memorial Dr.
Pocatello, ID 83201
208-232-6150

Magic Valley Memorial
Hospital
650 Addison Ave. W.
Twin Falls, ID 83301
208-737-2000

ILLINOIS

Children's Memorial Hospital
2300 Children's Plaza
Chicago, IL 60614
312-649-4000/4250

Cook County Hospital
1835 W. Harrison St.
Chicago, IL 60612
311-633-6000

Michael Reese Hospital
2929 S. Ellis Ave.
Chicago, IL 60616
312-791-2000

Northwestern Memorial
Hospital/Prentice Women's
Hospital
Superior St. and Fairbanks Ct.
Chicago, IL 60611
312-649-2000

Ravenswood Hospital
4550 N. Winchester Ave.
Chicago, IL 60640
312-878-4300

Rush-Presbyterian/St. Luke's
Medical Center
1753 W. Congress Pkwy.
Chicago, IL 60612
312-942-5000

St. Anthony Hospital
2875 W. Nineteenth St.
Chicago, IL 60623
312-521-1710

University of Chicago
Hospital and Clinics
Chicago Lying-In and Wyler
Children's Hospital
University of Chicago School
of Medicine
Chicago, IL 60637
312-947-1000

University of Illinois Hospital
1740 W. Taylor
Chicago, IL 60612
312-996-9634

St. Mary's Hospital
1800 E. Lake Shore Dr.
Decatur, IL 62525
217-429-2966

Memorial Hospital of DuPage County
200 Berteau Ave.
Elmhurst, IL 60126
312-833-1400

Evanston Hospital
2650 Ridge Ave.
Evanston, IL 60201
312-492-2000

Loyola University Medical Center
2160 S. First Ave.
Maywood, IL 60153
312-531-3000

Christ Hospital
4440 W. Ninety-fifth St.
Oak Lawn, IL 60453
312-425-8000

Lutheran General Hospital
1775 Dempster St.
Park Ridge, IL 60068
312-696-2210

Methodist Medical Center of Illinois
221 NE Glen Oak
Peoria, IL 61636
309-672-5522

St. Francis Hospital Medical Center
530 NE Glen Oak Ave.
Peoria, IL 61637
309-672-2000

Rockford Memorial Hospital
2400 N. Rocton Ave.
Rockford, IL 61101
815-968-6861

Memorial Medical Center
800 N. Rutledge St.
Springfield, IL 62781
217-788-3000

St. John's Hospital
800 E. Carpenter St.
Springfield, IL 72769
217-544-6464

Mercy Hospital
1400 W. Park
Urbana, IL 61801
217-337-2233

Central DuPage Hospital
O N. 025 Winfield Rd.
Winfield, IL 60190
312-682-1600

INDIANA

St. Francis Hospital Center
1600 Albany St.
Beechgrove, IN 46107
317-787-3311

Bartholomew County Hospital
2400 Seventeenth St.
Columbus, IN 47201
812-379-4441

St. Catherine Hospital of East Chicago
4321 Fir St.
East Chicago, IN 46312
219-392-1700

Elkhart General Hospital
600 East Blvd.
Elkhart, IN 46514
219-294-2621

St. Mary's Medical Center of Evansville
3700 Washington Ave.
Evansville, IN 47750
812-473-2100

Welborn Baptist Hospital
401 SE Sixth St.
Evansville, IN 47713
812-426-8000

Parkview Memorial Hospital
2200 Randalia Dr.
Fort Wayne, IN 46805
219-484-6636

St. Margaret Hospital
5424 Hohman Ave.
Hammond, IN 46320
219-932-2300

Community Hospital of
Indianapolis, Inc.
1500 N. Ritter Ave.
Indianapolis, IN 46219
317-353-1441

Indiana University Medical
Center
1100 W. Michigan St.
Indianapolis, IN 46223
317-635-8431

Methodist Hospital of Indiana
1604 N. Capitol St.
Indianapolis, IN 46202
317-924-6411

St. Vincent Hospital and
Health Care Center
2001 W. Eighty-sixth St.
Indianapolis, IN 46260
317-871-2345

William N. Wishard
Memorial Hospital
1001 W. Tenth St.
Indianapolis, IN 46202
317-639-6671

Lafayette Home Hospital
2400 South St.
Lafayette, IN 47903
317-447-6811

Reid Memorial Hospital
1401 Chester Blvd.
Richmond, IN 47374
317-962-4545

Memorial Hospital
615 N. Michigan Ave.
South Bend, IN 46601
219-234-9041

Union Hospital
1606 N. Seventh St.
Terre Haute, IN 47804
812-238-7000

Porter Memorial Hospital
814-818 LaPorte Ave.
Valparaiso, IN 46383
219-464-8611

IOWA

Mary Greeley Memorial
Hospital
117 Eleventh St.
Ames, IA 50010
515-239-2001

Burlington Medical Center
602 N. Third St.
Burlington, IA 52601
319-753-3011

St. Luke's Methodist Hospital
1026 A Ave. NE
Cedar Rapids, IA 52402
319-369-7211

St. Luke's Hospital
1227 E. Rusholme St.
Davenport, IA 52803
319-326-6512

Raymond Blank Memorial
Hospital for Children
Iowa Methodist Medical
Center
1200 Pleasant St.
Des Moines, IA 50308
515-283-6212

Mercy Health Center
St. Joseph Unit
Mercy Dr.
Dubuque, IA 52011
319-588-8400

Trinity Regional Hospital
S. Kenyon Rd.
Fort Dodge, IA 50501
515-573-3101

Mercy Hospital
500 Market St.
Iowa City, IA 52240
319-337-0500

University of Iowa Hospital
and Clinics
Newton Rd.
Iowa City, IA 52242
319-356-1616

St. Joseph Mercy Hospital
Sisters of Mercy Health Corp.
84 Beaumont Dr.
Mason City, IA 50401
515-424-7211

St. Luke's Medical Center
2720 Stone Park Blvd.
Sioux City, IA 51104
712-279-3500

St. Francis Hospital
3421 W. Ninth St.
Waterloo, IA 50702
319-236-4111

KANSAS

Dodge City Regional Hospital
3001 Ave. A
Dodge City, KS 67801
316-225-9050

Newman Memorial County
Hospital
Twelfth and Chestnut St.
Emporia, KS 66801
316-343-6800

Irwin Army Community
Hospital
Fort Riley, KS 66442
913-239-7101

Mercy Hospital
821 Burke St.
Fort Scott, KS 66701
316-223-2200

St. Catherine Hospital
608 N. Fifth St.
Garden City, KS 67846
316-275-6111

St. Anthony Hospital
Canterbury Rd.
Hays, KS 67601
913-625-7301

Hutchinson Hospital Corp.
1701 E. Twenty-third St.
Hutchinson, KS 67501
316-663-6811

Bethany Medical Center
51 N. Twelfth St.
Kansas City, KS 66102
913-281-8400

University of Kansas College
of Health Sciences
Bell Memorial Hospital
Thirty-ninth St. and Rainbow
Blvd.
Kansas City, KS 66103
913-588-5000

Memorial Hospital
Sunset Ave. and Chaflin Rd.
Box 1208
Manhattan, KS 66502
913-776-3300

Asbury Hospital
400 S. Santa Fe Ave.
Box 1608
Salina, KS 67401
913-827-4411

Shawnee Mission Medical
Center
Seventy-fourth and Grandview
St.
Box 2923
Shawnee Mission, KS 66201
913-676-2000

Stormont-Vail Regional
Medical Center
1500 W. Tenth St.
Topeka, KS 66606
913-354-6000

St. Francis Hospital of
Wichita
929 N. St. Francis Ave.
Box 1358
Wichita, KS 67201
316-268-5000

St. Joseph Medical Center
3600 E. Harry St.
Wichita, KS 67218
316-685-1111

Wesley Medical Center
550 N. Hillside
Wichita, KS 67214
316-688-2360

KENTUCKY

King's Daughters' Hospital
2200 Lexington Ave.
Ashland, KY 41101
606-329-2133

Medical Center at Bowling
Green
250 Park St.
Box 56
Bowling Green, KY 42101
502-781-2150

Southeastern Kentucky
Baptist Hospital
Mitchell St.
Corbin, KY 40701
606-528-1212

St. Elizabeth Medical Center-
North
401 E. Twentieth St.
Covington, KY 41014
606-292-4000

St. Luke Hospital of Campbell
County
85 N. Grand Ave.
Fort Thomas, KY 41075
606-292-3100

T. J. Samson Community
Hospital
N. Jackson Hwy.
Box 257
Glasgow, KY 42141
502-651-6171

Community Methodist
Hospital
1305 N. Elm St.
Box 48
Henderson, KY 42420
502-826-6251

Jennie Stuart Memorial
Hospital
Hospital Lane
Hopkinsville, KY 42240
502-886-5221

Central Baptist Hospital
1740 S. Limestone
Lexington, KY 40503
606-278-3411

University of Kentucky Medical Center
800 Rose St.
Lexington, KY 40536
606-233-5000

Audubon Hospital
1 Audubon Plaza
Louisville, KY 40217
502-636-7111

Kosair Children's Hospital, Medical Center, NKC, Inc.
200 E. Chestnut St.
P.O. Box 35070
Louisville, KY 40232
502-589-8000

Methodist Evangelical Hospital
315 E. Broadway St.
Box 843
Louisville, KY 40202
502-585-2241

St. Anthony Hospital
1313 St. Anthony Pl.
Louisville, KY 40204
502-587-1161

University Hospital
550 S. Jackson St.
Louisville, KY 40202
502-588-7000

Regional Medical Center
Hospital Dr.
Madisonville, KY 42431
502-825-5100

St. Clair Medical Center
Medical Circle
Morehead, KY 40351
606-784-6661

Western Baptist Hospital
2501 Kentucky Ave.
Paducah, KY 42001
502-444-5100

Methodist Hospital of Kentucky
US 23 By-pass
Pikeville, KY 41501
606-437-9621

Lake Cumberland Medical Center
305 Langdon St.
Box 620
Somerset, KY 42501
606-679-7441

LOUISIANA

Women's Hospital
9050 Airline Hwy.
Baton Rouge, LA 70815
504-927-1300

East Jefferson General Hospital
4200 Houma Blvd.
Metairie, LA 70011
504-454-4000

Lakeside Hospital
4700 Interstate 10
Metairie, LA 70001
504-885-3333

Charity Hospital of Louisiana
1532 Tulane Ave.
New Orleans, LA 70140
504-523-2311

Ochsner Foundation Hospital
1516 Jefferson Hwy.
New Orleans, LA 70121
504-838-3000

Southern Baptist Hospital
2700 Napoleon Ave.
New Orleans, LA 70175
504-899-9311

Tulane Medical Center
Hospital and Clinics
1415 Tulane Ave.
New Orleans, LA 70112
504-588-5471

Louisiana State University
Hospital
1541 Kings Hwy.
Box 33932
Shreveport, LA 71130
318-674-5000

Schumpert Medical Center
915 Margaret Pl.
Box 21976
Shreveport, LA 71120
318-227-4215

Willis-Knighton Medical
Center
2600 Greenwood Rd.
Shreveport, LA 71103
318-227-4600

MAINE

Maine Medical Center
22 Bramhall St.
Portland, ME 04102
207-871-0111

MARYLAND

Baltimore City Hospital
4940 Eastern Ave.
Baltimore, MD 21224
301-396-9067

John Hopkins Hospital
600 N. Wolfe St.
Baltimore, MD 21205
301-955-5000

St. Agnes Hospital
Wilkens and Caton Ave.
Baltimore, MD 21229
301-368-6000

Sinai Hospital of Baltimore
Belvedere and Greenspring
Ave.
Baltimore, MD 21215
301-578-5216

University of Maryland
Hospital
22 S. Greene St.
Baltimore, MD 21201
301-528-6294

National Naval Medical
Center
8901 Wisconsin Ave.
Bethesda, MD 20814
301-295-2206

MASSACHUSETTS

Beth Israel Hospital
330 Brookline Ave.
Boston, MA 02115
617-735-2000

Boston City Hospital
818 Harrison Ave.
Boston, MA 02118
617-424-5000

Brigham and Women's
Hospital
75 Francis St.
Boston, MA 02115
617-732-5500

Children's Hospital Medical
Center
300 Longwood Ave.
Boston, MA 02115
617-735-6000

Massachusetts General
Hospital
32 Fruit St.
Boston, MA 02114
617-726-2000

St. Margaret's Hospital for Women
90 Cushing Ave.
Boston, MA 02125
617-436-8600

Framingham Union Hospital
115 Lincoln St.
Framingham, MA 01701
617-879-7111

Lawrence General Hospital
One General St.
Lawrence, MA 01842
617-683-4000

Baystate Medical Center Wesson Women's Unit
759 Chestnut St.
Springfield, MA 01107
413-787-3200

New England Memorial Hospital
5 Woodlawn Rd.
Stoneham, MA 02180
617-665-1740

Memorial Hospital
119 Belmont St.
Worcester, MA 01605
617-793-6611

MICHIGAN

University Hospital
1405 E. Ann St.
Ann Arbor, MI 48109
313-763-4109

Children's Hospital of Michigan
3901 Beaubien
Detroit, MI 48201
313-494-5301

Harper-Grace Hospital
3990 John R St.
Detroit, MI 48201
3313-494-9015

Henry Ford Hospital
2799 W. Grand Blvd.
Detroit, MI 48202
313-876-2600

Hutzel Hospital
4707 St. Antoine
Detroit, MI 48201
313-494-7171

Mt. Carmel Mercy Hospital of Sisters of Mercy Health Corp.
6071 W. Outer Dr.
Detroit, MI 48235
313-927-7088

St. John Hospital
22101 Moross Rd.
Detroit, MI 48236
313-343-4000

Sinai Hospital of Detroit
6767 W. Outer Dr.
Detroit, MI 48235
313-493-6824

Hurley Medical Center
1 Hurley Plaza
Flint, MI 48502
313-766-0000

Butterworth Hospital
100 Michigan NE
Grand Rapids, MI 49503
616-774-1774

Bronson Methodist Hospital
252 E. Lovell St.
Kalmazoo, MI 49007
616-383-7654

Edward W. Sparrow Hospital
1215 E. Michigan Ave.
Lansing, MI 48909
517-487-6111

Marquette General Hospital
420 W. Magnetic St.
Marquette, MI 49855
906-228-9440

Northern Michigan Hospital, Inc.
416 Connable Ave.
Petoskey, MI 49770
616-347-7373

Pontiac General Hospital
Seminole at W. Huron St.
Pontiac, MI 48053
313-857-7200

Port Huron Hospital
1001 Kearney St.
Port Huron, MI 48060
313-987-5000

William Beaumont Hospital Corp.
3601 Thirteen Mile Rd.
Royal Oak, MI 48067
313-288-1000

Saginaw General Hospital
1447 N. Harrison St.
Saginaw, MI 48602
517-771-4000

Providence Hospital
16001 W. Nine Mile Rd.
Southfield, MI 48075
313-424-3000

Munson Medical Center
Sixth and Madison
Traverse City, MI 49684
616-947-6140

Riverside Osteopathic Hospital
150 Truax St.
Trenton, MI 48183
313-676-4200

Wayne County General Hospital
2345 Merriman Rd.
Westland, MI 48185
313-274-3000

MINNESOTA

Mercy Medical Center
4050 Coon Rapids Blvd.
Coon Rapids, MN 55433
612-427-2200

St. Mary's Hospital
407 E. Third St.
Duluth, MN 55805
218-726-4000

Fairview Southdale Hospital
6401 France Ave. S.
Edina, MN 55435
612-920-4400

Unity Hospital
550 Osborne Rd. NE
Fridley, MN 55432
612-786-2200

Immanuel St. Joseph's Hospital
325 Garden Blvd.
Mankato, MN 56001
507-625-4031

Abbott-Northwestern Hospital
2727 Chicago Ave.
Minneapolis, MN 55407
612-874-4000

Children's Health Center
2525 Chicago Ave. S.
Minneapolis, MN 55404
612-874-6122

Fairview Hospital
2312 S. Sixth St.
Minneapolis, MN 55454
612-371-6300

Hennepin County Medical Center
Metropolitan Medical Center
701 Park Ave. S.
Minneapolis, MN 55415
612-347-2338

Methodist Hospital
6500 Excelsior Blvd.
St. Louis Park
Box 650
Minneapolis, MN 55440
612-932-5000

North Memorial Medical Center
3220 Lowry Ave. N.
Minneapolis, MN 55422
612-588-0616

St. Cloud Hospital
1406 Sixth Ave.
Minneapolis, MN 56301
612-251-2700

St. Mary's Hospital
2414 S. Seventh St.
Minneapolis, MN 55454
612-338-2229

University of Minnesota Hospital
420 Delaware St. SE
Minneapolis, MN 55455
612-373-8484

St. Mary's Hospital of Rochester
Rochester Methodist Hospital
1216 Second St. SW
Rochester, MN 55905
507-284-2511

Midway Hospital
1700 University Ave.
St. Paul, MN 55104
612-641-5500

St. Joseph's Hospital
69 W. Exchange St.
St. Paul, MN 55105
612-291-3000

St. Paul Ramsey Medical Center
640 Jackson
St. Paul, MN 55101
612-221-3456

United Hospital
333 N. Smith St.
St. Paul, MN 55102
612-298-8888

Rice Memorial Hospital
301 Becker Ave. SW
Willmar, MN 56201
612-235-4543

MISSISSIPPI

USAF Medical Center
Kessler Air Force Base
Biloxi, MS 39534
601-377-6012

Hinds General Hospital
1850 Chadwick Dr.
Jackson, MS 39204
601-376-1370

University of Mississippi Medical Center
University Hospital
2500 N. State St.
Jackson, MS 39216
601-987-3500

The Woman's Hospital
P.O. Box 4546
Jackson, MS 39216
601-932-1000

Singing River Hospital
2809 Denny Rd.
Pascagoula, MS 39567
601-938-5000

MISSOURI

Southeast Missouri Hospital
1701 Lacey St.
Cape Girardeau, MO 63701
314-334-4822

Boone County Hospital
1600 E. Broadway
Columbia, MO 65201
314-875-4545

University of Missouri Hospital and Clinics
807 Stadium Rd.
Columbia, MO 65212
314-882-3984

St. Elizabeth's Hospital
109 Virginia St.
Box 551
Hannibal, MO 63401
314-221-0414

Freeman Hospital
1102 W. Thirty-second St.
Joplin, MO 64801
417-623-2801

Children's Mercy Hospital
Twenty-fourth and Gillham Rd.
Kansas City, MO 64108
816-234-3000

Research Medical Center
2316 E. Meyer Blvd.
Kansas City, MO 64132
816-276-4000

St. Luke's Hospital
Wornall Rd. and Forty-fourth St.
Kansas City, MO 64111
816-932-2036

Truman Medical Center
2301 Holmes St.
Kansas City, MO 64108
816-556-3000

University of Health Sciences University Hospital
2105 Independence Blvd.
Kansas City, MO 64124
816-283-2000

Kirksville Osteopathic Health Center
800 W. Jefferson St.
Kirksville, MO 63501
816-626-2121

Methodist Medical Center
Seventh to Ninth on Faraon
St. Joseph, MO 64501
816-271-7111

Barnes Hospital
499 S. Euclid
St. Louis, MO 63110
314-454-2000

Cardinal Glennon Memorial Hospital for Children
1465 S. Grand Blvd.
St. Louis, MO 63104
314-577-5600

Jewish Hospital of St. Louis
216 S. Kings Highway Blvd.
Box 14109
St. Louis, MO 63178
314-454-7000

Lutheran Medical Center
2639 Main St.
St. Louis, MO 63118
314-772-1456

St. John's Mercy Medical Center
615 S. New Ballas Rd.
St. Louis, MO 63141
314-569-6000

St. Louis Children's Hospital
500 S. Kings Highway Blvd.
St. Louis, MO 63178
314-367-6880

St. Mary's Health Center
6420 Clayton Rd.
St. Louis, MO 63117
314-768-8000

Lester E. Cox Medical Center
1423 N. Jefferson St.
Springfield, MO 65802
417-836-3000

St. John's Regional Health Center
1235 E. Cherokee St.
Springfield, MO 65802
417-885-2000

MONTANA

St. Vincent Hospital
Box 2505
Billings, MT 59103
406-657-7000

St. James Community Hospital
400 S. Clark St.
Butte, MT 59701
406-792-8361

Montana Deaconess Medical Center
1101 Twenty-sixth St. S.
Great Falls, MT 59405
406-761-1200

Kalispell Regional Hospital
310 Sunnyview Lane
Kalispell, MT 59901
406-755-5111

Holy Rosary Hospital
2101 Clark St.
Miles City, MT 59301
406-232-2540

Missoula Community Hospital
2827 Fort Missoula Rd.
Missoula, MT 59801
406-728-4100

NEBRASKA

St. Francis Medical Center
2620 W. Faidley Ave.
Box 2118
Grand Island, NE 68801
308-384-4600

Mary Lanning Memorial Hospital
715 N. St. Joseph Ave.
Hastings, NE 68901
402-463-4251

St. Elizabeth Community Health Center
555 S. 70th St.
Lincoln, NE 68510
402-489-7181

Great Plains Medical Center
601 W. Leota St.
Box 1167
North Platte, NE 69101
308-534-9310

Archbishop Bergan Mercy Hospital
7500 Mercy Rd.
Omaha, NE 68124
402-398-6060

Children's Memorial Hospital
8301 Dodge St.
Omaha, NE 68114
402-390-3000

St. Joseph's Hospital
601 N. 30th St.
Omaha, NE 68131
402-449-4000

University of Nebraska Medical Center
Forty-second and Dewey Ave.
Omaha, NE 68105
402-559-4000

West Nebraska General
Hospital
4021 Ave. B
Scottsbluff, NE 69361
308-635-3711

NEVADA

Sunrise Hospital Medical
Center
3186 Maryland Pkwy.
Las Vegas, NV 89109
702-731-8000

St. Mary's Hospital
235 W. Sixth St.
Reno, NV 89503
702-323-2041

Washoe Medical Center
77 Pringle Way
Reno, NV 89520
202-785-4100

NEW HAMPSHIRE

Dartmouth-Hitchcock Medical
Center
2 Maynard St.
Hanover, NH 03755
603-643-4000

NEW JERSEY

Atlantic City Medical Center
1925 Pacific Ave.
Atlantic City, NJ 08401
609-344-4081

Clara Maass Memorial
Hospital
Franklin Ave.
Bellville, NJ 07109
201-751-1000

Cooper Medical Center
One Cooper Plaza
Camden, NJ 08103
609-342-2000

Our Lady of Lourdes Medical
Center
1600 Haddon Ave.
Camden, NJ 08103
609-757-3500

John F. Kennedy Medical
Center
James St.
Edison, NJ 08818
201-321-7000

Elizabeth General Hospital
and Dispensary
925 E. Jersey St.
Elizabeth, NJ 07201
201-289-8600

St. Elizabeth Hospital
225 Williamson St.
Elizabeth, NJ 07207

Englewood Hospital
350 Engle St.
Englewood, NJ 07631
201-894-3000

Hackensack Hospital
Hospital Pl.
Hackensack, NJ 07601
201-487-4000

St. Mary Hospital
308 Willow Ave.
Hoboken, NJ 07030
201-383-2121

Jersey City Medical Center
50 Baldwin Ave.
Jersey City, NJ 07304
201-451-9800

St. Barnabas Medical Center
Old Short Hills Rd.
Livingston, NJ 07039
201-533-5000

Monmouth Medical Center
300 Second Ave.
Long Branch, NJ 07740
201-222-5200

Morristown Memorial Hospital
100 Madison Ave.
Morristown, NJ 07960
201-540-5000

Burlington County Memorial Hospital
175 Madison Ave.
Mount Holly, NJ 08060
609-267-0700

Jersey Shore Medical Center/ Fitkin Hospital
1945 Corlies Ave.
Neptune, NJ 07753
201-775-5500

Middlesex General Hospital
180 Somerset St.
New Brunswick, NJ 08901
201-828-3000

St. Peter's Medical Center
254 Easton Ave.
New Brunswick, NJ 08903
201-745-8600

Children's Hospital of New Jersey
College Hospital
New Jersey Medical School
15 S. Ninth St.
Newark, NJ 07107
201-268-8000

Newark Beth Israel Medical Center
201 Lyons Ave.
Newark, NJ 07112
201-926-7203

United Hospital of Newark
15 S. Ninth St.
Newark, NJ 07107
210-268-8000

Newton Memorial Hospital
175 High St.
Newton, NJ 07860
201-383-2121

Passaic General Hospital
350 Boulevard
Passaic, NJ 07055
201-365-4568

Barnert Memorial Hospital Center
680 Broadway
Paterson, NJ 07514
201-684-8000

St. Joseph's Hospital and Medical Center
703 Main St.
Paterson, NJ 07503
201-977-2000

Perth Amboy General Hospital
530 New Brunswick Ave.
Perth Amboy, NJ 08861
201-442-3700

Muhlenberg Hospital
Park Ave. and Randolph Rd.
Box 1272
Plainfield, NJ 07061
201-668-2000

Riverview Hospital
35 Union St.
Red Bank, NJ 07701
201-741-2700

Valley Hospital
Linwood and N. Van Dien
Ave.
Ridgewood, NJ 07451
201-445-4900

Somerset Medical Center
Rehill Ave.
Somerville, NJ 08876
201-725-4000

John F. Kennedy Memorial
Hospital–Stratford Division
18 E. Laurie Rd.
Stratford, NJ 08084
609-784-4000

Overlook Hospital
193 Morris Ave.
Summit, NJ 07901
201-522-2000

Rancocas Valley Hospital
Sunset Rd.
Willingboro, NJ 08046
609-877-6000

Underwood Memorial
Hospital
N. Broad St. and Red Bank
Ave.
Woodbury, NJ 08096
609-845-0100

NEW MEXICO

Lovelace Medical Center
5400 Gibson Blvd. SE
Albuquerque, NM 87108
505-842-7073

Presbyterian Hospital
1100 Central SE
Albuquerque, NM 87102
505-841-1234

University of New Mexico
Hospital
Bernalillo County Medical
Center
2211 Lomas Blvd. NE
Albuquerque, NM 87106
505-843-2111

San Juan Regional Medical
Center
801 W. Maple St.
Farmington, NM 87401
505-325-5011

Memorial General Hospital
Telshor and University St.
Las Cruces, NM 88001
505-522-8641

Eastern New Mexico Medical
Center
405 W. Country Club Dr.
Roswell, NM 88201
505-622-8170

St. Vincent Hospital
455 St. Michaels Dr.
Box 2107
Santa Fe, NM 87501
505-983-3361

NEW YORK

Albany Medical Center
Hospital
43 New Scotland Ave.
Albany, NY 12208
518-445-5582

St. Peter's Hospital
315 S. Manning Blvd.
Albany, NY 12208
518-454-1550

Bronx Municipal Hospital Center
Albert Einstein College of Medicine
1300 Morris Park Ave.
Bronx, NY 10461
212-430-5000

New York Medical College
Lincoln Hospital Center
234 E. 149th St.
Bronx, NY 10451
212-579-5000

Brookdale Hospital Medical Center
Linden Blvd. at Brookdale Plaza
Brooklyn, NY 11212
212-240-5000

Brooklyn Hospital
121 DeKalb Ave.
Brooklyn, NY 11201
212-270-4411

Jewish Hospital Medical Center of Brooklyn
555 Prospect Pl.
Brooklyn, NY 11238
212-240-1000

Kings County Hospital Center
Downstate Medical Center
451 Clarkson Ave.
Brooklyn, NY 11203
212-735-3131

Maimonides Medical Center
4802 Tenth Ave.
Brooklyn, NY 11219
212-270-7679

Children's Hospital of Buffalo
219 Bryant St.
Buffalo, NY 14222
716-878-7000

Mercy Hospital
565 Abbott Rd.
Buffalo, NY 14220
716-826-7000

Arnot-Ogden Memorial Hospital
Roe Ave. and Grove St.
Elmira, NY 14901
607-737-4100

Flushing Hospital and Medical Center
Parsons Blvd. and Forty-fifth Ave.
Flushing, NY 11355
212-670-5000

Long Island Jewish–Hillside Medical Center
75-59 263rd St.
Glen Oaks, NY 11004
212-470-2000

Women's Christian Association Hospital
207 Foote Ave.
Jamestown, NY 14701
716-487-0141

United Health Services– Wilson Hospital
33-57 Harrison St.
Johnson City, NY 13790
607-773-6000

North Shore University Hospital
300 Community Dr.
Manhasset, NY 11030
516-562-0100

Nassau Hospital
259 First St.
Mineola, NY 11501
516-663-0333

Bellevue Hospital Center
First Ave. and Twenty-seventh St.
New York, NY 10016
212-561-4141

Mount Sinai Hospital
1 Gustave L. Levy Pl.
New York, NY 10029
212-650-6500

New York Medical College Metropolitan Hospital Center
1901 First Ave.
New York, NY 10029
212-360-6797

New York University Medical Center
400 E. Thirty-fourth St.
New York, NY 10016
212-340-6200

Presbyterian Hospital in the City of New York
622 W. 168th St.
New York, NY 10032
212-694-2500

St. Vincent's Hospital and Medical Center of New York
153 W. Eleventh St.
New York, NY 10011
212-790-9000

Society of the New York Hospital
525 E. Sixty-eighth St.
New York, NY 10021
212-472-6874

Nyack Hospital
N. Midland Ave.
Nyack, NY 10960
914-358-6200

Rochester General Hospital
1425 Portland Ave.
Rochester, NY 14621
716-338-4000

Strong Memorial Hospital
601 Elmwood Ave.
Rochester, NY 14642
716-275-2121

St. Vincent's Medical Center of Richmond
355 Bard Ave.
Staten Island, NY 10310
212-390-1234

Crouse-Irving Memorial Hospital
736 Irving Ave.
Syracuse, NY 13210
315-424-6611

The House of the Good Samaritan
830 Washington St.
Watertown, NY 13601
315-785-4000

NORTH CAROLINA

Memorial Mission Hospital
509 Biltmore Ave.
Ashville, NC 28801
704-255-4000

North Caroline Memorial Hospital
Manning Dr.
Chapel Hill, NC 27514
919-966-4131

Charlotte Memorial Hospital and Medical Center
1000 Blythe Blvd.
Box 32861
Charlotte, NC 28232
704-373-2121

Duke University Hospital
Box 3708
Durham, NC 27710
919-684-2713

Cape Fear Valley Hospital
Owen Dr.
Box 2000
Fayetteville, NC 28302
919-323-6151

Moses H. Cone Memorial Hospital
1200 N. Elm St.
Greensboro, NC 27420
919-379-3900

Pitt County Memorial Hospital
East Carolina University Medical School
P.O. Box 6028
Greenville, NC 27834
919-757-4100

Wake County Medical Center
3000 New Bern Ave.
Raleigh, NC 27610
919-755-8000

Forsyth Memorial Hospital
3333 Silas Creek Pkwy.
Winston-Salem, NC 27103
919-773-3000

North Carolina Baptist Hospital
300 S. Hawthorne Rd.
Winston-Salem, NC 27103
919-727-4051

NORTH DAKOTA

St. Alexius Hospital
Ninth and Thayer Ave.
Bismarck, ND 58501
701-224-7000

Dakota Hospital
1720 University Dr. S.
Fargo, ND 58103
701-280-4100

St. Luke's Hospital
Fifth St. N. at Mills Ave.
Fargo, ND 58122
701-280-5000

United Hospital
1200 Columbia Rd. S.
Grand Forks, ND 58201
701-780-5000

Trinity Medical Center
Burdick Expressway at Main St.
Minot, ND 58701
701-857-5000

OHIO

Akron City Hospital
525 E. Market St.
Akron, OH 44309
216-375-3000

Children's Hospital Medical Center of Akron
281 Locust St.
Akron, OH 44302
216-379-8200

Aultman Hospital
2600 Sixth St. SW
Canton, OH 44710
216-452-9911

Timkin Mercy Medical Center
1320 Timkin Mercy Dr. NW
Canton, OH 44708
216-489-1000

Bethesda Hospital
619 Oak St.
Cincinnati, OH 45206
513-559-6000

Cincinnati General Hospital
234 Goodman St.
Cincinnati, OH 45267
513-872-3100

Good Samaritan Hospital
3217 Clifton Ave.
Cincinnati, OH 45220
513-872-1400

University of Cincinnati
Children's Hospital Medical
Center
231 Bethesda Ave.
Cincinnati, OH 45267
513-872-5341

Cuyahoga County Hospital
3395 Scranton Rd.
Cleveland, OH 44109
216-398-6000

Fairview General Hospital
18101 Lorain Ave.
Cleveland, OH 44111
216-476-7000

Mt. Sinai Hospital of
Cleveland
University Circle
Cleveland, OH 44106
216-421-4000

St. Luke's Hospital of the
United Methodist Church
11311 Shaker Blvd.
Cleveland, OH 44104
216-368-7000

University Hospital of
Cleveland
Rainbow Babies' and
Children's Hospital
2074 Abington Rd.
Cleveland, OH 44106
216-444-1000

Children's Hospital
700 Children's Dr.
Columbus, OH 43205
614-461-2000

Grant Hospital
309 E. State St.
Columbus, OH 43215
614-461-3232

Mount Carmel Medical
Center
793 W. State St.
Columbus, OH 43222
614-225-5000

Riverside Methodist Hospital
3535 Olentangy River Rd.
Columbus, OH 43214
614-261-5000

University Hospital
410 W. Tenth Ave.
Columbus, OH 43210
614-421-8660

Children's Medical Center
One Children's Plaza
Dayton, OH 45404
513-226-8300

Good Samaritan Hospital and
Health Center
2222 Philadelphia Dr.
Dayton, OH 45405
513-278-2612

Grandview Hospital
405 Grand Ave.
Dayton, OH 45402
513-226-3200

Miami Valley Hospital
One Wyoming St.
Dayton, OH 45409
513-223-6192

St. Elizabeth Medical Center
601 Miami Blvd.
Dayton, OH 45408
513-223-3141

Elyria Memorial Hospital
630 E. River St.
Elyria, OH 44035
216-323-3221

Kettering Medical Center
3535 Southern Blvd.
Kettering, OH 45429
513-298-4331

Community Hospital of Springfield and Clark County
2615 E. High St.
Box 1228
Springfield, OH 45501
513-325-0531

Riverside Hospital
1600 Superior St.
Toledo, OH 43601
419-729-5151

St. Vincent Hospital and Medical Center
2213 Cherry St.
Toledo, OH 43608
419-259-4089

Toledo Hospital
2142 N. Cove Blvd.
Toledo, OH 43606
419-473-4218

Trumbull Memorial Hospital
1350 E. Market St.
Warren, OH 44482
216-841-9011

USAF Medical Center
Wright Patterson Air Force Base, OH 45433
513-257-6154

Greene Memorial Hospital
1141 N. Monroe Dr.
Xenia, OH 45385
513-372-8011

St. Elizabeth Medical Center
1044 Belmont Ave.
Box 1790
Youngstown, OH 44501
216-746-7211

Tod Babies' and Children's Hospital
500 Gypsy Lane
Youngstown, OH 44501
216-747-1431

Youngstown Hospital Association
345 Oak Hill Ave.
Youngstown, OH 44501
216-747-0751

OKLAHOMA

Mercy Health Center
4300 W. Memorial Rd.
Oklahoma City, OK 73120
405-751-3050

Oklahoma Children's Memorial Hospital
940 NE Thirteenth St.
Box 26307
Oklahoma City, OK 73126
405-271-6165

Oklahoma Memorial Hospital
800 NE Thirteenth St.
Oklahoma City, OK 73104
405-271-4700

St. Francis Hospital Eastern Oklahoma Perinatal Center
6161 S. Yale
Tulsa, OK 74177
918-494-2200

St. John's Medical Center
1923 S. Utica Ave.
Tulsa, OK 74104
918-744-2345

OREGON

St. Charles Medical Center
2500 NE Neff Rd.
Bend, OR 97701
503-382-4321

Good Samaritan Hospital
360 NW Samaritan Dr.
Box 1068
Corvallis, OR 97330
503-757-5111

Sacred Heart General
Hospital
1200 Alder St.
Box 10905
Eugene, OR 97440
503-686-7300

Rogue Valley Memorial
Hospital
2825 Barnett Rd.
Medford, OR 97501
503-773-6281

Bess Kaiser Medical Center
5055 N. Gruley Ave.
Portland, OR 97217
503-285-9321

Emanuel Hospital
2801 N. Gantenbein Ave.
Portland, OR 97227
503-280-3200

Good Smaritan Hospital &
Medical Center
1015 NW Twenty-second Ave.
Portland, OR 97210
503-229-7711

Portland Adventist Medical
Center
10123 SE Market
Portland, OR 97216
503-239-6150

University of Oregon Health
Sciences Center
3181 SW Sam Jackson Park
Rd.
Portland, OR 97201
503-225-8311

Salem Hospital–General Unit
2561 Center St. NE
Box 14001
Salem, OR 97309
503-370-5200

PENNSYLVANIA

Abington Memorial Hospital
1200 York Rd.
Abington, PA 19001
215-885-4000

Allentown Hospital
Association
Seventeenth and Chew St.
Allentown, PA 18102
215-821-2204

Altoona Hospital
Howard Ave. and Seventh St.
Altoona, PA
814-946-2011

Mercy Hospital
2500 Seventh Ave.
Altoona, PA 16603
814-944-1681

Delaware Valley Medical
Center
Wilson Ave. and Pond St.
Bristol, PA 19007
215-245-2200

Bryn Mawr Hospital
Bryn Mawr Ave.
Bryn Mawr, PA 19010
215-896-3000

Gesinger Medical Center
Danville, PA 17822
717-275-6211

Mercy Catholic Medical Center
Fitzgerald Mercy Division
Lansdown Ave. and Baily Rd.
Darby, PA 19023
215-237-4000

Maple Ave. Hospital
Maple Ave.
DuBois, PA 15801
814-371-3440

Hamot Medical Center
201 State St.
Erie, PA 16550
814-455-6711

St. Vincent Health Center
232 W. Twenty-fifth St.
Box 740
Erie, PA 16544
814-459-4000

Hanover General Hospital
Highland Ave. and Charles St.
Hanover, PA 17331
717-637-3711

Harrisburg Hospital
S. Front St.
Harrisburg, PA 17101
717-782-3131

Polyclinic Medical Center
Third St. and Polyclinic Ave.
Harrisburg, PA 17110
717-782-4141

St. Joseph Hospital
687 N. Church St.
Hazelton, PA 18201
717-459-4444

The Milton S. Hershey Medical Center
500 University Dr.
Hershey, PA 17033
717-534-8521

Indiana Hospital
P.O. Box 788
Indiana, PA 15701
412-357-7000

Conemagh Valley Memorial Hospital
1086 Franklin St.
Johnstown, PA 15905
814-536-6671

Lee Hospital
320 Main St.
Johnstown, PA 15901
814-535-7541

Lancaster General Hospital
555 N. Duke St.
Box 3555
Lancaster, PA 17603
717-299-5511

Lancaster Osteopathic Hospital
1175 Clark St.
Box 3002
Lancaster, PA 17604
717-397-3711

St. Joseph Hospital
250 College Ave.
Box 3509
Lancaster, PA 17604
717-291-8211

Lock Haven Hospital and
Extended Care Unit
24 Cree Dr.
Lock Haven, PA 17745
717-748-7721

Sacred Heart Hospital
1430 DeKalb St.
Norristown, PA 19401
215-275-4000

Albert Einstein Medical
Center
Northern Division
York and Tabor Rds.
Philadelphia, PA 19141
215-456-6010

Chestnut Hill Hospital
8835 Germantown Ave.
Philadelphia, PA 19118
215-248-8200

Children's Hospital of
Philadelphia
Thirty-fourth St. and Civic
Center Blvd.
Philadelphia, PA 19104
215-596-9100

Frankford Hospital of the
City of Philadelphia
Knights and Red Lion Rds.
Philadelphia, PA 19114
215-831-2000

Hahnemann Medical College
and Hospital
230 N. Broad St.
Philadelphia, PA 19102
215-448-7000

Hospital of the Medical
College of Pennsylvania
3300 Henry Ave.
Philadelphia, PA 19129
215-842-6000

Hospital of Philadephia
College of Osteopathic
Medicine
4150 City Ave.
Philadelphia, PA 19131
215-581-6000

Hospital of the University of
Pennsylvania
3400 Spruce St.
Philadelphia, PA 19104
215-662-4000

Lankenau Hospital
Lancaster Ave. W. of City
Line
Philadelphia, PA 19151
215-645-2000

Nazareth Hospital
2601 Holme Ave.
Phildelphia, PA 19152
215-335-6000

Pennsylvania Hospital
Eighth and Spruce St.
Philadelphia, PA 19107
215-829-3000

St. Christopher's Hospital for
Children
2600 N. Lawrence St.
Philadelphia, PA 19122
215-427-5000

The Salvation Army Booth
Maternity Center
6051 Overbrook Ave.
Philadelphia, PA 19131
215-878-7800

Temple University Hospital
3401 N. Broad St.
Philadelphia, PA 19140
215-221-2000

Thomas Jefferson University Hospital
Eleventh and Walnut St.
Philadelphia, PA 19107
215-928-6000

Allegheny General Hospital
320 E. North Ave.
Pittsburgh, PA 15212
412-237-3131

Children's Hospital of Pittsburgh
125 DeSota St.
Pittsburgh, PA 15213
412-647-2345

Magee Women's Hospital
Forbes Ave. and Halket St.
Pittsburgh, PA 16213
412-647-2345

Mercy Hospital of Pittsburgh
1400 Locust St.
Pittsburgh, PA 15219
412-232-8111

St. Francis General Hospital
Forty-fifth St. off
Pennsylvania Ave.
Pittsburgh, PA 15201
412-622-4343

Western Pennsylvania Hospital
4800 Friendship Ave.
Pittsburgh, PA 15224
412-578-5000

Reading Hospital and Medical Center
Sixth Ave. and Spruce St.
Reading, PA 19603
215-378-6000

St. Joseph Hospital
215 N. Twelfth St.
Box 316
Reading, PA 19603
215-378-2000

Community Medical Center
1822 Mulberry St.
Scranton, PA 18510
717-961-6161

Mercy Hospital
746 Jefferson Ave.
Scranton, PA 18501
717-348-7100

The Williamsport Hospital
777 Rural Ave.
Williamsport, PA 17701
717-322-7861

York Hospital
1001 S. George St.
York, PA 17405
717-771-2345

RHODE ISLAND

Women and Infants Hospital
50 Maude St.
Providence, RI 02908
401-274-1100

SOUTH CAROLINA

Medical University Hospital of South Carolina
171 Ashley Ave.
Charleston, SC 29403
803-792-3131

Naval Regional Medical Center
Charleston, SC 29408
803-743-6699

Richland Memorial Hospital
3301 Harden St.
Columbia, SC 29203
803-765-7011

Greenville Hospital System
701 Grove St.
Greenville, SC 29605
803-242-7000

Spartansburg General
Hospital
101 E. Wood St.
Spartansburg, SC 29303
803-573-6200

SOUTH DAKOTA

Sioux Valley Hospital
1001 S. Euclid Ave.
Sioux Falls, SD 57105
605-336-3440

TENNESSEE

Baroness Erlanger Hospital
975 E. Third St.
Chattanooga, TN 37403
615-755-7011

T. C. Thompson Children's
Hospital
910 Blackford St.
Chattanooga, TN 37403
615-755-6011

University of Tennessee
Memorial Hospital
1924 Alcoa Hwy.
Knoxville, TN 37920
615-971-3011

Baptist Hospital East
6019 Walnut Grove Rd.
Memphis, TN 38119
901-766-5000

E. H. Crump Women's
Hospital & Perinatal Center
853 Jefferson
Memphis, TN 38163
901-528-7835

Methodist Hospital Central
1265 Union Ave.
Memphis, TN 38104
901-726-7491

Vanderbilt University Medical
Center
Twenty-first and Garland
Nashville, TN 37232
615-322-7311

Oak Ridge Hospital of the
United Methodist Church
125 W. Tennessee Ave.
Box 529
Oak Ridge, TN 37830
615-482-2441

TEXAS

Hendrick Medical Center
Nineteenth and Hickory St.
Abilene, TX 79601
915-677-3551

Amarillo Hospital District
Northwest Texas Hospital
2200 W. Seventh St.
Amarillo, TX 79106
806-376-4431

Brackenridge Hospital
Fifteenth St. and East Ave.
Austin, TX 78701
512-476-6461

St. David's Community
Hospital
919 E. Thirty-second St.
Box 4039
Austin, TX 78765
512-476-7111

Seton Medical Center
1201 W. Thirty-eighth St.
Austin, TX 78705
512-835-0025

St. Elizabeth Hospital
2830 Calder Ave.
Box 5405
Beaumont, TX 77702
713-892-7171

**Driscoll Foundation
Children's Hospital**
3533 S. Alameda St.
Corpus Christi, TX 78411
512-854-5341

Memorial Medical Center
2606 Hospital Blvd.
Corpus Christi, TX 78405
512-884-4100

Spohn Hospital
1436 Third St.
Corpus Christi, TX 78404
512-884-2041

**Baylor University Medical
Center**
3500 Gaston Ave.
Dallas, TX 75246
214-820-0111

**Children's Medical Center of
Dallas**
1935 Amelia St.
Dallas, TX 75235
214-637-3820

Methodist Hospital of Dallas
Box 22599
Dallas, TX 75265
214-944-8181

Parkland Memorial Hospital
5201 Harry Hines Blvd.
Dallas, TX 75235
214-637-8000

Presbyterian Medical Center
8200 Walnut Hill Lane
Dallas, TX 75231
214-369-4111

St. Paul Hospital
5909 Harry Hines Blvd.
Dallas, TX 75235
214-689-2000

**Providence Memorial
Hospital**
2001 N. Oregon St.
El Paso, TX 79902
915-542-6011

**R. E. Thomason General
Hospital**
4815 Alameda Ave.
El Paso, TX 79905
915-544-1200

Sierra Medical Center
1625 Medical Center Dr.
El Paso, TX 79902
915-532-4000

**William Beaumont Army
Medical Center**
Piedras St.
El Paso, TX 79920
915-569-2201

**Darnall Army Community
Hospital**
Fort Hood, TX 76544
817-685-3110

**Fort Worth Children's
Hospital**
400 Cooper St.
Fort Worth, TX 76104
817-336-9861

Harris Hospital–Methodist
1300 W. Cannon St.
Fort Worth, TX 76104
817-334-6011

Tarrant County Hospital
District
John Peter Smith Hospital
1500 S. Main St.
Fort Worth, TX 76104
817-921-3431

University of Texas Medical
Branch Hospital
Eighth and Mechanic St.
Galveston, TX 77550
713-765-1011

Hermann Hospital
1203 Ross Sterling Ave.
Houston, TX 77025
713-797-4011

Jefferson Davis Hospital
1801 Allen Pkwy.
Houston, TX 77019
713-751-8000

St. Joseph Hospital
1919 La Branch
Houston, TX 77002
713-757-1000

St. Luke's Episcopal Hospital
6720 Bertner Ave.
Houston, TX 77025
713-791-2011

Texas Children's Hospital
6621 Fannin St.
Houston, TX 77030
713-791-2831

Woman's Hospital of Texas
7600 Fannin St.
Houston, TX 77054
713-790-1234

Lubbock County Hospital
District
Lubbock General Hospital
602 Indiana Ave.
Box 5980
Lubbock, TX 79417
806-743-3111

McAllen Methodist Hospital
701 S. Main St.
McAllen, TX 78501
512-687-7611

Pasadena Bayshore Hospital
4000 Spencer Hwy.
Pasadena, TX 77504
713-944-6666

Brooke Army Medical Center
San Antonio, TX 78234
512-221-3225

Medical Center Hospital
The University of Texas
Health Science Center
7703 Floyd Curl Dr.
San Antonio, TX 78284
512-691-7118

Santa Rosa Medical Center
519 W. Houston St.
San Antonio, TX 78285
512-228-2011

Southwest Texas Methodist
Hospital
7700 Floyd Curl Dr.
San Antonio, TX 78229
812-696-1200

Wilford Hall USAF Medical
Center
San Antonio, TX 78236
512-670-7351

Hays Memorial Hospital
Highway 35 N.
Box 767
San Marcos, TX 78666
512-392-3324

Scott and White Memorial Hospital
2401 S. Thirty-first St.
Temple, TX 76508
817-774-2111

Wadley Hospital
1000 Pine St.
Box 1878
Texarkana, TX 75501
214-793-4511

UTAH

Logan Regional Hospital
1400 N. 500 E.
Logan, UT 84321
801-752-2050

Cottonwood Hospital
5770 S. 300 E.
Murray, UT 84107
801-262-3461

McKay-Dee Hospital Center
3939 Harrison Blvd.
Ogden, UT 84409
801-627-2800

St. Benedict's Hospital
5475 S. Adams
Ogden, UT 84403
801-479-2111

Utah Valley Hospital
1034 N. 500 W.
Provo, UT 84601
801-373-7850

Holy Cross Hospital
1045 E. 100 S.
Salt Lake City, UT 84102
801-350-4111

Latter Day Saints Hospital
325 Eighth Ave.
Salt Lake City, UT 84143
801-350-1100

Primary Children's Medical Center
320 Twelfth Ave.
Salt Lake City, UT 84103
801-363-1221

University of Utah Medical Center
50 N. Medical Dr.
Salt Lake City, UT 84132
801-581-2680

VERMONT

Medical Center Hospital of Vermont
Colchester Ave.
Burlington, VT 05401
802-656-2345

VIRGINIA

Johnston Memorial Hospital
Court St.
Abingdon, VA 24210
703-628-3121

Alexandria Hospital
4320 Seminary Rd.
Alexandria, VA 22304
703-379-3000

University of Virginia Hospital
Jefferson Park Ave.
Charlottesville, VA 22908
804-924-0211

Memorial Hospital
142 S. Main St.
Danville, VA 24541
804-799-2100

The Fairfax
Hospital
3300 Gallows Rd.
Falls Church, VA 22046
703-698-1110

Virginia Baptist Hospital
3300 Rivermont Ave.
Lynchburg, VA 24503
804-384-4000

Memorial Hospital of
Martinsville and Henry
County
Commonwealth Blvd.
Box 4788
Martinsville, VA 24112
703-632-2911

Riverside Hospital
J. Clyde Morris Blvd.
Newport News, VA 23601
804-599-2000

Children's Hospital of the
King's Daughters
800 W. Olney Rd.
Norfolk, VA 23507
804-628-3000

Depaul Hospital
150 Kingsley Lane
Norfolk, VA 23505
804-489-5000

Norfolk General
Hospital
600 Gresham Dr.
Norfolk, VA 23508
804-628-3000

Naval Regional Medical
Center
Portsmouth, VA 23708
804-398-5111

Medical College of Virginia
Virginia Commonwealth
University
MCV Station Box 276
1200 E. Broad St.
Richmond, VA 23298
804-786-9965

Community Hospital of
Roanoke Valley
101 Elm Ave. SE
Box 12946
Roanoke, VA 24029
703-345-1031

Roanoke Memorial Hospital
Bellview at Jefferson St.
Box 13367
Roanoke, VA 24033
703-981-7000

Lewis-Gale Hospital
1900 Electric Rd.
Salem, VA 24153
703-989-4261

WASHINGTON

Harrison Memorial Hospital
2520 Cherry Ave.
Box 2077
Sheridan Park Station
Bremerton, WA 98310
206-377-3911

General Hospital of Everett
1321 Colby Ave.
Everett, WA 98201
206-258-6300

Monticello Medical Center
600 Broadway
Longview, WA 98632
206-423-5850

St. Peter Hospital
413 N. Lilly Rd.
Olympia, WA 98506
206-491-9480

Kadlec Hospital
888 Swift Blvd.
Richland, WA 99352
509-946-4611

Children's Orthopedic
Hospital and Medical Center
4800 Sand Point Way NE
Seattle, WA 98105
206-634-5000

Group Health Cooperative
Central Hospital
201 Sixteenth Ave. E.
Seattle, WA 98112
206-326-6262

Riverton General Hospital
12844 Military Rd. S.
Seattle, WA 98168
206-244-0180

Swedish Hospital Medical
Center
747 Summit Ave.
Seattle, WA 98104
206-292-2121

University of Washington
Hospital
1959 Pacific Ave. NE
Seattle, WA 98195
206-543-3010

Virginia Mason Hospital
925 Seneca St.
Box 1930
Seattle, WA 98111
206-624-1144

Deaconess Hospital
800 W. Fifth Ave.
Spokane, WA 99210
509-624-0171

Sacred Heart Medical Center
101 W. Eighth Ave.
Spokane, WA 99220
509-455-3131

Madigan Army Medical
Center
Tacoma, WA 98431
206-926-6817

Tacoma General Hospital
315 S. K St.
Tacoma, WA 98405
206-597-7700

St. Mary Community Hospital
401 W. Poplar St.
Box 1477
Walla Walla, WA 99362
509-525-3320

Yakima Valley Memorial
Hospital
2811 Tieton Dr.
Yakima, WA 98902
509-575-8000

WEST VIRGINIA

Charleston Area Medical
Center
Brooks St. and Elmwood Ave.
Charleston, WV 25325

United Hospital Center, Inc.
Route 19 S.
Box 1680
Clarksburg, WV 26301
304-624-2121

Cabell Huntington Hospital
1340 Hal Greer Blvd.
Huntington, WV 72501
304-696-6110

West Virginia University
Medical Center
Morgantown, WV 26506
304-293-4536

WISCONSIN

Luther Hospital
310 Chestnut St.
Eau Claire, WI 54701
715-839-3311

St. Vincent Hospital
835 S. Van Buren St.
Green Bay, WI 54305
414-432-8631

La Crosse Lutheran Hospital
1910 South Ave.
La Crosse, WI 54601
608-785-0530

Madison General Hospital
202 S. Park
Madison, WI 53715
608-267-6000

St. Mary's Hospital and Medical Center
707 S. Mills St.
Madison, WI 53715
608-251-6100

St. Joseph Hospital
611 St. Joseph Ave.
Marshfield, WI 54449
715-387-1713

Family Hospital
2711 W. Wells St.
Milwaukee, WI 53206
414-937-2100

Milwaukee Children's Hospital
1700 W. Wisconsin Ave.
Milwaukee, WI 53233
414-931-1010

Milwaukee County Medical Complex
8700 W. Wisconsin Ave.
Milwaukee, WI 53226
414-257-7900

Mt. Sinai Medical Center
950 N. Twelfth St.
Milwaukee, WI 53233
414-289-8001

St. Joseph's Hospital
5000 W. Chambers
Milwaukee, WI 53210
414-447-2000

Theda Clark Regional Medical Center
130 Second St.
Neenah, WI 54956
414-729-3100

WYOMING

Memorial Hospital of Natrona County
1233 E. Third St.
Casper, WY 82601
307-577-7201

Memorial Hospital of Laramie County
300 E. Twenty-third St.
Cheyenne, WY 82001
307-634-3341

Suggested Reading

(Based on recommendations from the University of California, San Francisco, prenatal care programs.)

Pregnancy and Birth

Ashdown-Sharp, Patricia. *A Guide to Pregnancy and Parenthood for Women on Their Own*, 1977; explores options in both practical and emotional terms; lists resources.

Bing, Elisabeth, and Colman, Libby. *Making Love During Pregnancy*, 1977; couples talk about sexual changes during pregnancy; illustrated with sensitive drawings.

Colman, Arthur and Libby. *Pregnancy, The Psychological Experience*, 1972; an analysis of the psychological states of all members of the "pregnant" family.

Isbister, Clair. *Birth of a Family, A Preparation for Parenthood*, 1975; the practical and medical aspects of pregnancy and childbirth.

Milinaire, Caterine, *Birth*, 1974; contains birth histories of numerous deliveries.

Nilsson, Lennart, et al. *A Child Is Born*, 1979; a dramatic pictorial revelation of human reproduction from conception to birth.

Childbirth Preparation

Bradley, Robert. *Husband-Coached Childbirth*, rev. 1974; Bradley method.

Ewy, Donna, and Ewy, Rodger. *Preparation for Childbirth*, rev. 1976; popular, well-illustrated Lamaze guide.

Miller, John. *Childbirth: A Manual for Pregnancy and Delivery*, rev. 1974; emphasizes learning total body relaxation.

Noble, Elizabeth. *Essential Exercises for the Childbearing Year*, 1976; therapeutic exercises for pregnancy and postpartum; includes cesarean rehabilitation; written by a physical therapist.

Cesarean Birth

Donovan, Bonnie. *The Cesarean Birth Experience*, 1977; guide to family-centered cesarean birth.

Breast-feeding

Eiger, Marvin, and Olds, Sally. *The Complete Book of Breastfeeding,* 1972; comprehensive, easy reading, includes a section on possible problems and solutions.

LaLeche League, International. *The Womanly Art of Breastfeeding,* 1963; a manual condensing the years of experience of LaLeche League mothers in helping others breast-feed.

Pryor, Karen, *Nursing Your Baby,* 1973; informative, with both technical information and a week-by-week description.

Books for Brothers and Sisters

Nilsson, Lennart. *How Was I Born?,* 1975; story of reproduction and birth for children; beautiful photographs.

Rushnell, Elaine Evans. *My Mom's Having a Baby,* 1978; based on the ABC Afterschool Special.

Sheffield, Margaret. *Where Do Babies Come From?,* 1973; explicit without being frightening; colored paintings.

Parenting and Child Development

Biller, Henry, and Meredith, Dennis. *Father Power,* 1974; effective fathering advice by two fathers.

Boston Women's Health Collective, *Ourselves, Our Children,* 1978; a book by and for parents; discusses parenting from consideration to parent to parenting grownups; also includes various family styles.

Briggs, Dorothy Corkille. *Your Child's Self Esteem,* 1975; the key to life; creating feelings of self-worth.

Burck, F. *Baby Sense,* 1979; a guide to baby care.

Dodson, Fitzhugh, *How to Parent,* 1970; a psychologist's guide; lots of specific advice on bowel training, discipline, and education.

Samuels, Mike and Nancy. *The Well Baby Book;* a holistic approach to pregnancy and children in health and disease; helps parents find their own solutions to the problems of raising children.

Spock, Benjamin, M.D. *Baby and Child Care,* updated edition; detailed discussion of the numerous physical and social problems from infancy to age five; large part of book devoted to well-baby care.

White, Burton. *The First Three Years of Life,* a guide to physical, emotional, and intellectual growth of your baby.

Women's Health

Barbach, Lonnie Garfield, *For Yourself,* 1975; step-by-step program of education regarding a woman's discovery of her sexuality.

Boston Women's Health Book Collective. *Our Bodies, Ourselves,* rev. 1976; factual, concise and open presentation of female bodily processes; covers puberty through childbirth; information on birth control.

Montague, Ashley. *Touching,* 1971; discusses how tactile experience, or its lack, affects the development of behavior.

Nutrition

Brewer, Gail, with Brewer, Tom. *What Every Pregnant Woman Should Know: The Truth About Diet and Drugs in Pregnancy,* 1977; discusses relation of nutrition and toxemia as well as good nutrition in pregnancy.

Williams, Phyllis. *Nourishing Your Unborn Child,* 1974; nutrition during pregnancy and postpartum plus menus and recipes.

Index